For Churchill Livingstone:

Senior Commissioning Editor: Ninette Premdas
Project Manager: Gail Murray
Project Development Manager: Katrina Mather
Designer: George Ajayi

Cancer Nursing Practice

A Textbook for the Specialist Nurse

Edited by

Nora Kearney MSc RGN
Senior Lecturer in Cancer Nursing, Nursing and Midwifery School, University of Glasgow, Glasgow, UK

Alison Richardson BN(Hons) MSc PhD RN PGDipEd RNT
Professor of Cancer and Palliative Nursing Care, The Florence Nightingale School of Nursing and Midwifery, King's College London, London, UK

Paola Di Giulio MSc RN
Nurse Researcher, Unità di Ricerca Infermieristica, Istituto Mario Negri, Milan, Italy

Foreword by

Ainna Fawcett-Henesy
Regional Advisor Nursing and Midwifery, World Health Organization, Regional Office for Europe, Copenhagen, Denmark

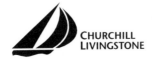

EDINBURGH LONDON NEW YORK PHILADELPHIA ST LOUIS SYDNEY TORONTO 2000

CHURCHILL LIVINGSTONE
An imprint of Harcourt Publishers Limited

© Harcourt Publishers Limited 2000

 is a registered trademark of Harcourt Publishers Limited

First published 2000

ISBN 0 443 06040 1

British Library Cataloguing in Publication Data
A catalogue record for this book is available from the British Library

Library of Congress Cataloging in Publication Data
A catalog record for this book is available from the Library of Congress

Note
Medical knowledge is constantly changing. As new information becomes available,
changes in treatment, procedures, equipment and the use of drugs become necessary.
The editors, contributors and the publishers have taken care to ensure that the
information given in this text is accurate and up to date. However, readers are
strongly advised to confirm that the information, especially with regard to drug
usage, complies with the latest legislation and standards of practice.

Printed in China

The
publisher's
policy is to use
**paper manufactured
from sustainable forests**

Contents

Contributors

Phyllis Campbell BSc RGN SCM
Nurse Manager, Beatson Oncology Centre, Western Infirmary, Glasgow, UK

Alison Ferguson BA(Hons) MSc RGN OCN PGDE
Programme Director – Practice Development, Centre for the Development of
Nursing Policy and Practice, University of Leeds, Leeds, UK

Agnes Glaus MSc PhD RN
Clinical Nurse Specialist, Centre for Tumour Detection and Prevention, St Gallen,
Switzerland

Carol R. Krcmar RN MN
Clinical Nurse Specialist Oncology, Private Practice, Stuttgart, Germany

Karin Magnusson MSc RN
Head of Unit, Unit of Research and Development, Department of Oncology,
Sahlgrenska University Hospital, Gothenberg, Sweden

Emma Ream BSc(Hons) MSc RN RGN
Lecturer in Nursing, The Florence Nightingale School of Nursing and Midwifery,
King's College London, London, UK

Kathy Redmond MSc RGN
Lecturer, School of Nursing and Midwifery, University College Dublin, Dublin,
Ireland

Lorraine Robinson BSc(Hons) MSc PGDE RGN
Principal Lecturer, The Florence Nightingale School of Nursing and Midwifery,
King's College London,
London, UK

P. Anne Scott BA(Hons) MSc PhD RGN
Senior Lecturer, Department of Nursing and Midwifery, University of Stirling,
Stirling, UK

Derek Waddell BA(Hons)
Deputy Director, Edinburgh Research and Innovation, University of Edinburgh,
Edinburgh, UK

Yvonne Willems-Cavalli RN
Consultant Oncology Nursing, Oncology Institute of Southern Switzerland (IOSI),
Bellinzona, Switzerland

Foreword

The World Health Organization's new health policy document for Europe, *Health 21*, identifies cancer as one of the major burdens of disease in Europe. It sets an ambitious target to which all countries should aspire: by the year 2020, morbidity, disability and premature mortality resulting from major chronic diseases should be reduced to the lowest feasible levels throughout the region. More specifically, it suggests that mortality resulting from cancers of all sites in people under 65 years should be reduced by at least 15% on average, and mortality resulting from lung cancer should be reduced by 25%.

Throughout this new health policy document nurses are singled out as having a key role to play throughout the whole continuum of care. In particular, nurses are seen as working with individuals, families and communities to promote health and prevent ill health as well as to care for people when they are ill. Supporting those in the terminal stages of illness as well as their families and friends, and ensuring a peaceful and dignified death, are also perceived as important nursing functions.

Whilst the challenges presented to the nursing profession in this new WHO policy statement are formidable, nurses in the cancer specialty in Europe have already taken great strides in the direction proposed. Not only have they been leaders in the development of nursing as a clinical based specialty but they have joined together to facilitate the sharing of skills, knowledge and experience as well as the competencies that underpin these to ensure that those who work in the specialty are safe and competent. Cancer nurses have also been at the forefront of interdisciplinary working, having in many instances established true partnerships with physician colleagues. Moreover, they have reached out to nurses in countries less well developed than their own to ensure that patients with cancer and their families receive equitable care where possible.

As health care is forever changing, demands ever increasing and new techniques and technology constantly being introduced, nurses in cancer, more than most other specialties, must be aware of the need to constantly update their knowledge and skills to ensure that their practice is current and based on the best available evidence. By implication, this requires them to have access to new thinking in management education practice and research within their specialty as well as within the broader nursing and healthcare agenda. This timely publication should be able to help them to do just that, and will act as a useful reference for both those working within the specialty and the many nurses who work with patients and their families with cancer every day at home and work, in institutions and hospices. This book covers a whole range of topics of relevance, including the thorny issue of clinical decision making and the ethical issues that are faced by both patients and those who care for them on a regular basis. This publication also offers a rare insight into how the specialty has developed, sometimes against the odds, and may act as an inspiration to other groups of nurses attempting to develop their specialty in the interests of better patient care.

This publication is a welcome addition to the many books on cancer nursing, especially so because it focuses on cancer nursing in Europe and the European dimension, one of the first nursing publications to do so.

Ainna Fawcett-Henesy

Preface

There is an ever growing number of texts relating to the evolving specialty of cancer nursing. We believe this particular book to be unique in that it is the first European text to address topics of concern to nurses practising beyond the novice level in cancer nursing. The text presents a synthesis of important issues that underpin the practice of cancer nursing at an advanced level. *Cancer Nursing Practice: A Textbook for the Specialist Nurse* evolved from the editors' involvement in cancer nursing at both a national and European level and their roles as researchers, educators, managers and practitioners. As active members of the European Oncology Nursing Society we became acutely aware of the dearth of European texts that addressed the needs of European cancer nurses. Whilst there is an accumulation of information emanating from North America, such texts are not always culturally transferable to nursing care within Europe. In addition the majority of texts on cancer nursing that are available address the knowledge base fundamental to developing the practice of the novice cancer nurse but often fail to focus in any detail on aspects of relevance to the specialist practitioner, and hence do not include a wider appreciation of the possibilities and challenges of advanced cancer nursing care.

Themes central to this book reflect the emerging roles of the specialist nurse and include advanced practice, education, management and research. The text embraces key aspects that will be of particular interest to those either engaged in graduate or postgraduate studies or undergoing a period of preparation to enable them to practise at an advanced level.

The contributors were chosen because of their backgrounds in the different domains of cancer nursing and for their expert knowledge of the context of cancer nursing in Europe. The chapters have all been written or co-authored by recognized cancer nursing experts from across Europe who are collectively involved in shaping the future of the specialty across the continent.

The essence of cancer nursing lies in its ability to impact on the quality of survival of individuals with cancer. Chapter 1 provides a review of the forces that have shaped cancer nursing in Europe. Chapter 2 addresses the practice base of cancer nursing and explores the development, scope and means necessary to support professional practice. Chapter 3 has as its focus leadership and management, and covers both the economic and emotional cost of cancer nursing and concepts critical to the management of a cancer nursing service. The theoretical and practical aspects which surround clinical decision making form the content of Chapter 4. A critical analysis of the nursing process and of the main theories that try to explain decision making is presented. Chapter 5 presents an overview of cancer nursing education across Europe, stressing the disparity of educational opportunities offered to cancer nurses. The major future challenges related to continuing professional education, accreditation and the application of the future opportunities of information technology are also discussed. Integral to the development of the specialty is increasing the knowledge base from which to practise, and the concept and context of cancer nursing research are highlighted in Chapter 6. Information giving and patient education are major components of the nurse's role and these are debated in Chapter 7, where the research that evaluates the effectiveness of patient information is presented. Chapter 8 deals with some of the most fundamental questions surrounding human interaction: the balance between respect and autonomy and paternalism in health care. Examples are presented to explore basic assumptions generally held regarding both patients and practice. The text culminates with a chapter that examines the existing structure of cancer nursing services in Europe. It reviews factors both current and future that are likely to influence the nature of the specialty, and concludes with the suggestion that the development of a strategic framework might be a positive vehicle through which to move cancer nursing in Europe forward.

The editors would like to thank Alex Mathieson for his encouragement during the early stages of development; Gail Murray, who saw the book through to publication from the perspective of our publisher; and Alex Balsdon, who so rigorously copy-edited the manuscript. And finally, we would like to express our gratitude to the authors of the individual chapters who enthusiastically embraced our outline for their individual contributions, thus ensuring that our original ideas evolved into a text that we hope will serve the cancer nursing community across Europe.

Nora Kearney
Alison Richardson
Paola Di Giulio

Glasgow, London and Milan 2000

CHAPTER 1

Cancer nursing as a specialty

Carol R. Krcmar

INTRODUCTION

Scope of the cancer problem

As the new millennium approaches, we are still confronted with a disease about which comparatively little is known. Promising new treatments have not had a significant impact on cancer cure rates. Arduous efforts to increase public awareness of risk factors associated with the development of many cancers have not borne the intended results, as is evident, for example, in the steadily increasing incidence and death rate from lung cancer in both sexes. Costly procedures intended to detect cancer in its early stages, for example the early detection of breast cancer, have had only a slight influence on survival rates for this type of cancer in American women (Landis et al 1998).

Cancer is responsible for one quarter of all deaths within the geographical boundaries of the European Union (EU). Data from 1990 (Esteves et al 1993) indicate an annual rate of 1.3 million new cases and 840 000 deaths due to cancer in the EU. Cancer statistics gathered in the United States over the past 60 years prognosticate an optimistic outlook in terms of cancer survival rates. In the 1930s, about one in four Americans with cancer were alive 5 years after treatment; about four of ten Americans who got cancer in 1997 are expected to be alive 5 years after diagnosis. Demographic trends are having a significant impact on cancer care. As the average age of the population increases, so does the increase in mortality due to cancer: the incidence of cancer is increasing in persons over 50 years of age and the median age at which cancer is diagnosed is now 65 years (Enghofer 1997).

The scope of the cancer problem encompasses more than morbidity and mortality statistics. For many persons, the diagnosis of cancer is associated with negative stigmas such as pain, suffering and death. Patients with cancer are often reluctant to discuss their diagnosis, even with family members and close friends. Changes in physical appearance, often the hallmarks of cancer treatment side-effects, may deter patients from leaving secure surroundings, which can lead to social isolation. The hopes and disappointments incurred through cycles of treatment and waiting for diagnostic results, combined with the adjustments necessary to adapt to living with a chronic disease, all impose an exceptional stress on persons with even the most effective coping mechanisms.

The costs of cancer are high, both to the individual and to society. The US National Cancer Institute (NCI) estimates overall costs for cancer at $104 billion; $35 billion for direct medical costs and $12 billion in relation to the costs associated with lost productivity. It has been recommended (Enghofer 1997) that health economists study the sources and causes for escalating cancer costs and the relation of these costs to the quality of care. Not only healthcare reform issues but also European political issues, as well as changing demographics, highlight the need to find new ways to treat cancer and restore a reasonable level of functional health to persons who have had cancer.

It is this very battle with a complex disease that sets cancer apart from other modern-day illnesses. This disease, which can indeed at a microscopic level resemble the outstretched claws of a crab, affects both young and old, male and female. Its complexity and the many unanswered questions surrounding this disease demand that healthcare professionals, scientists and politicians devote attention and financial support to identifying the causes, finding a cure, and educating the public about cancer. It is the vast scope of the cancer problem that has influenced its evolution into a specialty in both nursing and medicine.

In this chapter, the development of cancer nursing as a specialty in Europe, including factors that contribute to and hinder this development, is discussed. Role development of the expert nurse in cancer care, position, tasks and responsibilities as well as common practice settings are outlined. At the end of the chapter, a brief description of the outlook for the future of the specialty is presented.

The specialty of cancer nursing

Cancer nursing is a unique specialty within the profession of nursing. Although many individual factors have influenced the development of the specialty, it is fair to state that identification of the need for specialist knowledge and the resulting development of educational programmes played the most significant roles. In 1986, Ash wrote in an editorial in *Cancer Nursing* that 'there have always been nurses to provide care but not with the specialty knowledge and skill required and so evident today' (p. A17). This statement remains relevant 13 years after it was written.

The specialty of cancer nursing came of age in a time when it was recognized that clinical experience alone was not satisfactory as a means to further knowledge (Yasko 1991). Formal education is needed. To provide quality care to patients with cancer and their families, nurses require a sound knowledge base in physiology, pharmacology, psychology and sociology. Formal education courses, shorter continuing education programmes, mentor–protégé relationships, government and community resources, as well as specialty journals, all promote learning (Cooley, Spatz & Yasko 1996).

Nursing is a practice discipline. The acquisition of skills and knowledge through clinical experience is essential to attain and maintain good clinical practice. Cancer nursing is a specialty that is distinguished by the challenge to incorporate new technological advances continuously into practice. One need only reflect on the state of cancer nursing 10 years ago to realize how significantly medical advances impact on nursing. The challenge of updating practice is coupled with the challenge to address the complex physical and emotional demands of patients (Whitley 1992). The complexity of cancer care stems from multimodal treatment, the intensity of treatment effects, and the number of professional disciplines and treatment settings that are involved.

As in other areas of care, nursing's contribution to cancer care exceeds the mere utilization of technical skills and application of specialist knowledge. In this high-tech area of healthcare, with emphasis on incidence, mortality and survival rates, nurses' contribution is a softer more emotion-focused type of therapy, which complements medical treatment (Corner 1997). Corner's description of this softer contribution of nurses to cancer care is supported by the results of a study conducted by Haberman et al (1994) which identified, among other items, the caring behaviours of oncology nurses. A sampling of the behaviours noted in this study included:

- being with patients
- preserving dignity at the time of death
- not giving up on patients
- maintaining hope
- minimizing suffering

- protecting patient privacy
- anticipating patient needs
- sharing self.

Nurses in the above-noted study also expressed frustration, especially at the failure of treatment. For many nurses, the disappointments and sorrow experienced when medical interventions fail to prolong life are counterbalanced by the value of the intrinsic rewards that come from helping individuals, no matter what the outcome. A philosophy of care that reflects the individual's own identified standard of professional practice can serve as a useful self-assessment tool when inner conflict arises between idealistic goals and limitations imposed by the reality of the situation.

Philosophy of cancer care

The development and implementation of an individual philosophy of care provides a framework to assist the nurse to focus activities. This personal philosophy must be in tangent with the philosophy of colleagues in the work setting, where a collective philosophy should be discussed, adjusted and refined to maintain its relevance. A central component of a philosophy of cancer care should be one of the features of therapeutic cancer nursing as described by Corner (1997). Corner proposes an integrated view of the patient; that is the acknowledgement of the inseparable nature of mind and body in the experience of cancer-related problems and needs. A holistic approach to addressing patient problems and needs, which, in addition to all aspects of the mind–body interaction also takes into account the social sphere of the individual, has long been embraced by nurses and is a distinguishing difference between our practice and that of other healthcare professionals. Additional components of a philosophy of cancer nursing as proposed by McCorkle et al (1996) should incorporate the importance of collaboration with members of the multidisciplinary team, the primacy of the patient and family as decision-maker, and the education and research responsibility of staff members.

The multiprofessional approach to cancer care ensures that each team member applies specialized knowledge and skills collectively to provide quality care. The individuals who compose the team may vary depending on setting. The success of the multiprofessional approach is dependent on each member recognizing the expertise of the others. Further, each member must be regarded as having equal input into decision-making and be respected and acknowledged for their input.

Reaching a consensus on a philosophy of care, within the multiprofessional team, and collectively implementing this philosophy to achieve a common goal can help to strengthen an *esprit de corps* in clinical areas. The sense of working as a team provides support during emotionally exhausting periods. Just as a common philosophy of care supports and provides a focus for individual members of the healthcare team, the transparency of this work ideology and its positive outcomes can surely be identified and experienced by patients and families.

Central to a philosophy that promotes individual-centred care is the belief that patients have a right to be informed about their disease and treatment and to be consulted regarding treatment decisions. It is easier to ensure that these rights are respected if the multiprofessional team is in agreement as to the importance of providing patients and families with both the type and amount of information that patients deem necessary. Patients should receive a clear and consistent message that their participation in decision-making is valued by all collaborating members of the team.

A philosophy of cancer nursing incorporates the importance of education and research responsibilities of the nursing staff. Updating and renewing knowledge, the dissemination of knowledge to more novice colleagues, as well as educating patients and families are inherent activities in the role of the cancer nurse. Similarly, research activities including the incorporation of research results into practice should be identified in a philosophy and the value of such apparent to all staff members.

Historically, nurses have had difficulty identifying and placing a value on their contribution to the care of patients (McCorkle et al 1996). While medicine can demonstrate its contribution to cancer treatment with statistical results, a philosophy of caring cannot easily be measured in terms of its effect on outcome nor publicly displayed in graphical format. The various phases of cancer, from prevention in the form of genetic counselling through to terminal and bereavement care, and the acknowledged role of nursing during these phases, presents nurses with an opportunity to assume the management of patient care activities, more so than in other diseases. At the core of nursing activities is caring. Although perhaps not sufficiently researched, the therapeutic effects of human compassion, which is an important component of caring, does impact on patient outcome. Patients, who may be regarded as the ultimate judge of care, often express their appreciation for the care they received and acknowledge the effect that caring made to their experience of cancer.

HISTORICAL DEVELOPMENT OF CANCER NURSING

Development of cancer nursing in the United States

The evolution of cancer nursing as a specialty in the US well preceded that in Europe. Both in the US and Europe, as nurses' clinical skills in the management of cancer-related symptoms continued to develop and refine, so did recognition of the importance of the role of the nurse in cancer care. As early as 1952, the National Cancer Institute in the United States initiated a pilot course in postbasic cancer nursing (Yarbro 1996). The goal of this course was to support and enhance clinical knowledge with theoretical knowledge about cancer prevention, cause and treatment. The rapid growth of cancer nursing was influenced by increased funding for cancer research; medical, scientific and technological advances; public interest in cancer; and general changes in the nursing profession (Yarbro 1996, p. 19).

Many factors directly and indirectly associated with nursing influenced the development of the specialty of cancer nursing. As described by McCorkle et al (1996), specialty groups arise from a focus on a specific disease; a specific kind of treatment; or a specific phase of treatment received (i.e. based on medical diagnosis and treatment regimens). Nurses working on wards with frequent admissions of patients with cancer became clinical experts in that area. It is questionable whether the specialty would have developed as strongly and intensely as it has, had it not been for the collective and collaborative efforts of these nurses working on designated cancer wards.

In addition, the growth of cancer nursing specialization paralleled the growth of specialization in nursing in other areas in the 1960s (Jacobs & Kreamer 1997). This evolution instigated a change in nursing roles from generalist nurse to oncology nurse to clinical nurse specialist or advanced practitioner. The first oncology nursing programme at the master's level was started in 1968 at the University of Pittsburgh within the medical–surgical nursing programme (Jacobs & Kreamer 1997). The availability of master's degree programmes and postbasic certificate courses, combined with the financial and personnel support provided by hospital administrations, helped to create an environment conducive to continuing education. The recognition of cancer as a significant health hazard prompted governments to support cancer research and education. Cancer nurses themselves profited from the professional identity and exposure provided by the establishment of the Oncology Nursing Society in 1975. Conferences supported by this organization offered a means to update knowledge and collaborate on strategies to manage the many physical and psychosocial effects of cancer.

Development of cancer nursing in Europe

Before going into greater detail about the historical development of cancer nursing in Europe and its evolution in individual countries, a brief history and description of the European Oncology Nursing Society (EONS) will be provided. The activities and accomplishments of EONS can be accredited with having had either direct or indirect influence on the development of the specialty of cancer nursing in Europe as well as in individual countries (see Box 1.1).

EONS, founded in 1984, is comprised of individual cancer nurses, oncology nursing societies, and institutions and agencies involved in cancer care. EONS has a membership of over 50 organizations, which in turn represent approximately 15 000 nurses in 25 European countries. Membership of EONS was extended to include individual oncology nurses in 1997. The goal of the Society is to promote and develop cancer nursing in countries throughout Europe, which will in turn improve the quality of care that patients with cancer receive. Educational, consultative and research activities of EONS are aimed toward the achievement of this goal (see Box 1.2). One of the most successful initiatives of EONS to date has been the development of a core curriculum for a postbasic course in cancer nursing. This curriculum has had a profound effect on the movement to educate specialist nurses in cancer in Europe and has recently been revised to reflect contemporary cancer nursing practice (EONS 1999). The project to revise the

---

■ **BOX 1.1   Key milestones in the development of cancer nursing in Europe**

1980s	Expansion in the number of continuing education courses in cancer nursing
1980–1985	First postbasic courses in cancer nursing offered in various European countries
1984	European Oncology Nursing Society (EONS) founded
1989	Consensus conference on core curriculum for a postbasic course in cancer nursing
1991	Dissemination of the EONS core curriculum for a postbasic course in cancer nursing
1993	EONS accepted as a full member of the Federation of European Cancer Societies (FECS)
1996	Action on Fatigue: a European educational and research initiative for oncology nurses; attended by 200 nurses, simultaneous translation available
1997	Launch of *Oncology Nurses Today* (EONS newsletter), published in nine languages
1998	First EONS spring convention
1998	Expansion of EONS activities into former Eastern block countries
1998	Distribution of the *European Journal of Oncology Nursing*, official publication of EONS
1999	Development of an accreditation scheme for cancer nursing educational programmes

■ **BOX 1.2   Activities of the European Oncology Nursing Society (EONS)**

- Collaboration with the Advisory Committee on Training in Nursing (ACTN) on developing recommendations on the training of nurses in the matter of cancer at a basic, postbasic and advanced level.
- Development and subsequent revision of a core curriculum for a postregistration course in cancer nursing and the attainment of panEuropean consensus on the content and implementation of the core curriculum (EONS 1991, 1999).
- Development of educational materials for use in national training courses on altered body image, emesis, pain, psychological disorders and infection (Cancer Care: Priorities for Nurses project, supported by Smith Kline Beecham Pharmaceuticals).
- PanEuropean implementation of the programme 'Learning to Live with Cancer' developed by Getrud Grahn.
- Implementation of the Action on Fatigue project, based on the Oncology Nursing Society's Fatigue Initiative in Research and Education (FIRE) project, which has educational and research components (supported by Janssen Cilag).
- Launch of the *European Journal of Oncology Nursing*, the official journal of EONS, published quarterly.
- Distribution of *Oncology Nurses Today*, a newsletter published four times per year in seven languages (supported by Bristol-Myers Squibb).
- Support of initiatives designed to increase collaboration and networking possibilities among cancer nurses in Europe, for example the European Cancer Conference (ECCO) and the EONS spring convention.
- Development of an educational programme for advancing oncology nursing practice and the formulation of standards against which to audit cancer nursing – a joint project with the European Quality Assurance Network (EUROQUAN).
- Development and implementation of a scheme for the accreditation for cancer nursing education courses.
- Presentation of EONS activities on the World Wide Web (www.cancereurope.org).
- Co-facilitator in WISECARE (Workflow Information Systems for European Nursing Care) funded by the European Commission. This project aims to identify the unique contribution of cancer nursing across Europe through the use of information technology, and involves five countries.
- Collaboration with European and international organizations to foster the status and advancement of cancer nursing in Europe.

curriculum was funded by the Europe Against Cancer programme of the European Commission.

The Society is governed by an advisory council and a board of directors. The working language of the Society is English, although every effort is made to provide translation services at educational programmes and to translate resource materials into all European languages. EONS has formed working relationships with the International Society for Nurses in Cancer Care (ISNCC), the Oncology Nursing Society (ONS, of the United States), various European nursing organizations and specialty groups, the Advisory Committee on Training in Nursing (ACTN) and the Standing Committee of Nurses of the EU (PCN).

An event of significance in terms of the evolution of cancer nursing in Europe was the acceptance of EONS as a full member of the Federation of European Cancer Societies (FECS) in 1993. The primary aim of FECS is to promote and coordinate collaboration between European professional societies active in various aspects of cancer management. The status of nursing varies considerably across Europe; therefore the acceptance of EONS as an equal member of a multidisciplinary and interdisciplinary organization was, and continues to be, an impetus for the gradual recognition of the role of cancer nursing in individual European countries. Through collaboration on educational and research initiatives, clinical oncologists and basic scientists have gained a greater understanding of the contributions that nurses make to cancer care.

State of cancer nursing practice 10–15 years ago

In an effort to obtain information on the historical development of cancer nursing in various European countries, a questionnaire was distributed to 17 representatives of cancer nursing organizations that are members of EONS. Ten questionnaires were returned (Belgium, Denmark, Germany, Greece, Italy, The Netherlands, Norway, Spain, Sweden and UK). The responses provide a general overview of the past and current state of cancer nursing in those countries, identification of factors that influenced the development of the specialty, and the establishment and accomplishments of cancer nursing organizations in the respective countries.

The description of the state of cancer nursing 10–15 years ago provided by the respondents illustrates the progress, accomplishments and achievements that have occurred in cancer nursing in Europe in a fairly short span of time. In relation to the practice of cancer nursing, most respondents acknowledged that cancer nursing was not recognized as a specialty in the early to mid 1980s in their respective countries. This was noted to be due to several factors including the limited number of designated cancer centres and the practice of nurses, which was more likely to take the form of physician's assistant than of specialist practitioner. The role of the nurse in identifying and intervening in patient problems such as adequate pain control and symptom management was underdeveloped. Many respondents indicated that nurses caring for patients with cancer at this time found it difficult to identify their role in the cancer care team.

State of cancer nursing education

As can be interpreted from the results of the questionnaire, the state of cancer nursing education 10–15 years ago was very different to that found today. Educational offerings were diverse, and directed at providing knowledge and skills required for a particular patient care situation. Respondents indicated that the safe handling of cytotoxic drugs was a topic of concern to nurses and was similarly offered in both short courses as well as more extended courses of up to 30 hours. There were no mechanisms in place to evaluate the objectives and effectiveness of these courses. The explosion in cancer nursing education began in the mid 1980s, although the majority of respondents noted that continuing education courses at this time were for the most part organized by physicians and content was medically oriented.

The first postbasic course in cancer nursing in Denmark started in 1980, in 1982 in Norway, and in 1986 in Sweden. These courses well preceded the EONS consensus work on a postbasic course in cancer nursing, which was completed in 1991. National cancer nursing congresses began to appear in the mid- to late 1980s. The general dissemination of knowledge and practice methods as well as the beginning of networking among cancer nurses is attributed to the organization of these congresses. The impetus for the increased awareness of the need for continuing education included providing better care, keeping up with medical advances, and attaining practice standards of the calibre published in the international nursing literature.

Persons and forces that influenced the development of cancer nursing

Respondents were asked to identify the persons and/or organizations that helped to influence the development of cancer nursing in their respective countries. In the UK, for example, the targeting of cancer as a significant health problem by successive governments was noted to have a positive impact on the development and recognition of cancer nursing. In Spain, as early as 1982, nurses served as consultants to the department of health, therefore affecting change through political pathways. In Italy, increased public awareness of cancer and the public's demand for better cancer services influenced the development of nurses' education in cancer care.

Respondents acknowledged the support of the national nursing organization in encouraging the organization of cancer nursing groups. Interest in membership in national cancer nursing societies and/or cancer nursing interest groups of larger national nursing societies steadily increased over the next 10 years (the Dutch Oncology Nursing Society currently has a membership of 1500, the Norwegian Society boasts 1200 members). Other organizations credited with encouraging the development of cancer nursing and financially supporting educational initiatives included national cancer societies and regional comprehensive cancer centres. In Norway, Sweden and Spain the advancement of cancer nursing was identified as being linked to general advances in nursing education; that is the movement to educate nurses at the university level.

While not the case in many countries, two respondents noted that medical oncologists facilitated and encouraged the further education of nurses in cancer care. Outstanding nursing leaders were also identified as individuals who had strongly influenced the development of cancer nursing through networking, leadership and personal style. Robert Tiffany, one noted nursing leader, believed that nurses could dramatically change the care patients received and that skilled nurses played a crucial role in the prevention and early detection of cancer and in improving the quality of life for people with cancer (Delleport 1997). His influence was clearly felt not only in the UK, but in the international development of cancer nursing globally.

Persons and forces preventing the development of cancer nursing

Generally, a lack of resources, both individual and financial, were cited as impeding the development of cancer nursing. Before the initiation of postbasic cancer nursing courses, there was a paucity of qualified nurse educators in most European countries. Insufficient financial resources for the implementation of nursing research, identified by two respondents, has and will most likely continue adversely to affect further study of the effects of nursing interventions on patient outcome. More worrisome is the lack of recognition of the capabilities of nurse researchers to conduct scientific inquiry. Interestingly, both hospital administrators and labour unions were cited as resisting forces. Hospital administrators were unwilling to support cancer nursing advancement because of the increased salary costs associated with the hiring of specialist nurses (i.e. nurses with advanced degrees). In one country, labour unions were identified as resisting forces to the development of cancer nursing due to their expressed concern that the intensity of caring exclusively for patients with cancer would increase the risk of burnout in nurses.

Further, both individual nurses and national nursing organizations were identified as resistors to the development of cancer nursing. Individuals were sceptical about the general concept of specialization and were noted to be uncertain about the role of nurses in the cancer care team. Nursing organizations, although for the most part identified as supportive of cancer nursing, were also noted to be concerned about the further fractionation of patient care which could occur through specialization. One respondent commented that clinical nurses did not view the national nursing organization in that particular country as being helpful or influential in terms of cancer nursing.

Not surprisingly, three respondents identified physicians as well as other health-care professionals as resistant factors to the further development of cancer nursing. Reasons for their resistance included feeling threatened by nurses' increased knowledge and not accepting nursing's role in the multidisciplinary team. Four respondents clearly indicated that there were no known persons or forces that pre-vented the development of cancer nursing as a specialty in their country.

Development and accomplishments of national cancer nursing organizations

All 10 respondents identified the existence of either a national oncology nursing society or a national oncology nursing group existing as a subgroup of the national nursing organization in their country. Several noted that, although growth of the organization was at first slow and tedious due in part to insufficient financial sup-port, steady growth has occurred over the past 10 years. All organizations are ori-ented toward promoting the professional development of their members through continuing education opportunities either in the form of short courses, congresses or professional publications. From the descriptions given of the acceptance of these activities, it is evident that standards of care and other types of practice guidelines issued by these societies are well received and highly regarded by institutions and individual nurses.

Improved communication and networking possibilities between nurses in vari-ous healthcare settings have been facilitated through the activities of their soci-eties. The promotion of the organization of cancer nurses at the regional and local levels was also listed as a goal of some of these societies. While all societies target nurses as the main focus of their activities, the cancer nursing society in Spain also provides education to the general public about cancer prevention. The respondent from the Danish society noted that the provision of services to members is made possible in part through contributions made by pharmaceutical companies. The Norwegian society uses some of its financial resources to offer scholarships for nurses to attend conferences. The cumulative efforts of these organizations have no doubt served to increase recognition and awareness of the role of qualified nurses in improving the care of patients with cancer.

THE EXPERT CANCER NURSE

Role development

The essential component to the development of expert cancer nurses is a sound general nursing knowledge base. Nursing is a practice discipline; the theoretical base of this practice incorporates ideas and concepts from disciplines outside, but of relevance to, nursing, such as communication science, psychology and even organizational behaviour. These related disciplines serve to enhance, enrich and support the practice of nursing, and modern-day practice without the inclusion of such topics would be incomprehensible. The importance of basic nurse education will be discussed elsewhere in this book.

Although educational training and practice of nurses in Europe may differ from country to country, universal concepts of professionalism provide a common guide-line for the development of the role of the expert cancer nurse. Cooley, Spatz & Yasko (1996) stress that concepts of professionalism should be introduced early in career development and maintained throughout. These concepts are that cancer nurses are responsible for:

- achieving and maintaining competence in their specialty area
- advancing the practice of cancer nursing
- advocating the specialty of cancer nursing to colleagues, other health professionals, consumers and the general public.

To implement these concepts, the cancer nurse must acquire a knowledge and a practice base in cancer nursing (Cooley, Spatz & Yasko 1996). In today's healthcare environment, it is imperative that the specialist nurse keeps abreast of the issues currently affecting cancer care and future trends in areas such as healthcare economics, policy-making and population demographics, which continue to influence the profession and practice of cancer nursing. As Yasko (1991) writes: 'experience, coupled with a sound knowledge base, is the best teacher' (p. 24). Role development as an expert cancer nurse requires rich and varied clinical experiences which build on one another. Reflection and evaluation of these past experiences gleans knowledge that the expert uses further to advance practice.

Tasks and responsibilities

The number and variety of roles that cancer nurses can assume is broad. The most traditional and most common, of course, is direct patient care in facilities providing acute care. Tasks performed in this role include assessment, care planning, implementation, evaluation of interventions, documentation, collaboration with other healthcare professionals, and counselling patients and family. In addition to these tasks, the advanced cancer nurse has the responsibility to update knowledge regularly to reflect new advances in cancer, educate new members of staff, remain astute of management, administrative and political issues that directly or indirectly affect patient care, and conduct, utilize and evaluate research results for their applicability to patient care. A list of learned and acquired skills essential to the advanced cancer nurse are detailed in Table 1.1.

Table 1.1 Learned and acquired skills of cancer nurses

Skill	Application
Physical assessment and psychosocial assessment	Early recognition of complications Evaluation of interventions
Communication	Present patient needs Intercede as patient advocate Liaise with multidisciplinary team and other settings Make transparent the role of the cancer nurse
Time management	Establishment of priorities Completion of work in a timely manner Flexibility to accommodate the unexpected
Leadership	Mentor newer staff members Strengthen team cohesiveness Provide direction for team activities
Attention to detail	Prevention of errors (e.g. in chemotherapy)
Work independently	Assume responsibility for actions Adherence to professional standards

Nurses, by virtue of the amount of time spent with patients and the intensity of their interactions, are well suited to be the managers of the total care of patients. This involves not only administering direct care but also soliciting and coordinating the expertise of other members of the multiprofessional team. Patient care planning discussions, at which all disciplines are represented, reveal the multifaceted needs of patients and the interconnectiveness of those needs. The nurse assumes the role of patient advocate in the team while serving as contact person for the members of that team. As acute hospital stays shorten and patients are referred to specialists or specialty clinics, collaboration between nurses offering cancer care services in various settings must be established and maintained to ensure continuity of services.

Teaching is an important aspect of the expert cancer nurses' role. Teaching can be directed at patients and families, at new staff members, colleagues not regularly involved in cancer nursing, the public at large and healthcare professionals. The goals of teaching initiatives involving patients and families are to increase self-care activities, support decision-making and foster adaptation to changes in lifestyle (see Chapter 7).

Cancer nurses should assume a leadership role in educating the public about health promotion, cancer prevention and early detection, including the early warning signs of malignancy. Similarly, nurses should act as role models setting a good example by maintaining health through balanced nutrition, regular exercise and not smoking.

Expert cancer nurses may function in a primarily managerial role. Although not actively involved in direct patient care, nurse managers ensure the provision of services. Their roles include: maintaining and attaining quality assurance practices, policy making, initiating and evaluating cost containment measures, management of personnel, and strategic planning.

Cancer nurses have had a long history of involvement with research. This involvement entailed caring for patients enrolled in research treatment protocols and, as the specialty continued to develop, nurses participated in medical clinical trials as either data collectors or project managers. Patient contact with these clinical trial nurses varies according to the expectations of the principal investigator of the study. These nurses are often responsible for educating nursing staff about experimental treatments and their anticipated side-effects, as well as providing information about the implications of the clinical study that are pertinent to nursing practice. Nurses in advanced practice are responsible for disseminating research results and initiating changes in practice based on these results. Nurse researchers are beginning to participate as co-investigators in medical clinical trials studies, focusing their inquiry on quality of life issues. Priorities for cancer nursing research, as identified in an ONS survey include: pain, cancer prevention, quality of life, risk reduction and cancer screening, and ethical issues (Stetz et al 1995).

Practice settings

It is safe to assume that, at present in Europe, the majority of nurses involved in the provision of specialist care to patients with cancer are employed in acute care institutions and involved in direct patient care activities. Acute care facilities can be comprehensive cancer centres or community hospitals. Although hospital care is the most traditional place of employment for nurses, today they are involved in the provision of care at all stages of the disease trajectory in a variety of settings. The fastest growing area of employment opportunity is ambulatory care. Examples of ambulatory clinics are departments of hospitals, free-standing walk-in cancer clinics, or an office of a medical oncologist in private practice. The types of services offered include, but are not limited to: cancer treatment, uncomplicated diagnostic and palliative surgical procedures, follow-up examinations, symptom management and counselling services.

Boyle, Engelking & Harvey (1994) predict that home- and community-based care will be the norm in the twenty-first century. Roles of cancer nurses practising in ambulatory care include direct patient care, counselling, education, administrative tasks and liaison with colleagues and other healthcare providers. While care provided to patients at home once entailed supportive measures and terminal care, new technologies in medicine and telecommunications have opened the way for more intensive and complex treatments to be safely administered in this setting.

Changes are also occurring in rehabilitative care. Whereas patients were once admitted to rehabilitation clinics for physical and occupational therapy, measures aimed at optimizing physical and psychosocial functioning are provided by a multi-disciplinary team of healthcare professionals in the patient's home. Watson (1996) identifies the oncology advanced practice nurse specialist as a core member of this team. Nurses continue to be the key providers of hospice and palliative care services in the home setting. While not widespread in Europe, community agencies and industrial companies offer potential practice settings for expert cancer nurses who are capable of providing health promotion education and cancer screening services.

Expert cancer nurses

Expertise, as defined by Benner (1984), is necessary to be a specialist. Expertise is developed when the clinician tests and refines propositions, hypotheses and principle-based expectations in actual practice situations (Benner 1984). The expert gains experience when preconceived notions are challenged, refined and validated in actual clinical situations.

The most commonly implemented role of the expert is as practitioner. Whitley (1992) identified several characteristics of the expert oncology nurse. These experts, with their enormous background of patient care experience enhanced with postbasic education, are able quickly to assess a clinical situation and accurately target problems without time-consuming deliberation (Benner 1984). For example, expert nurses can quickly identify clinical problems or assess complex situations. Cancer nursing experts are attributed with intervening quickly and skilfully to prevent serious complications.

Finely tuned assessment skills can replace dependency on technological aids. Knowledge of the disease trajectory, expected treatment side-effects and general patient status allows the expert nurse in the acute care setting to predict patient needs and begin preparation for discharge care at an early stage.

The expert's influence on, and contribution to, quality care are many. The expert's practice often results in early and aggressive interventions. Ideally, the expert reduces the need for diagnostic tests and technological monitoring, prevents patient complications, provides early detection and reversal of complications, and alleviates patient complaints (Hanneman 1996). Because of the expert's ability to view the patient's care in its entirety, rather than be concerned with separate elements of care, the expert is better able to analyse the interrelationship between responses and interventions.

According to Hanneman (1996), society expects nurses to be more feeling oriented in decision-making rather than logical, analytical and unemotional. The presence of these characteristics, however, could compromise expert care in terms of the role of the nurse as patient advocate. As such, the nurse is expected to be objective, capable of confrontation and able to utilize facts as a basis for discussion and decision-making. A nurse expert in pain management uses the entire patient picture as it relates to pain control and not the usual parameters (Whitley 1992).

Patients experiencing pain quickly gain trust in the nurse expert who combines knowledge of pharmacology with clinical experience and effective communication skills to design an effective pain management regimen.

One way in which the finely tuned knowledge and skills acquired by experts can be disseminated is through consultancy. Wright (1992) acknowledges that nurses may have had, and continue to experience, difficulty labelling and marketing their expert competence as consultative work. Consultant nurses are not impinging on any other professional's domain nor are they expecting undue prestige when they offer their expertise to correct identified inadequacies. Four types of consultant activity are identified by Caplan (1970):

1. Nurse-centred (an expert nurse provides advice to a general nurse).
2. Patient-centred (the consultant advises other nurses on patient care management).
3. Programme-centred (planning staff development programmes).
4. Administration-centred (providing advice to administration on nursing policy and practice).

Crucial to the success of the consultant role of the expert cancer nurse is organizational recognition and support.

The expert cancer nurse is an asset to patient care and a resource for cancer nurses. These nurses are valuable members of the healthcare team. The complexity of care makes the interchangeability and easy replacement of expert nurses expensive and incongruent with quality of care (Benner 1984). Therefore, administrators must explore ways to keep expert nurses at the bedside. Retention of these nurses may be enhanced through better salaries, increased participation in important decision-making, and formal recognition of responsibility and achievements (Benner 1984). Clinical advancement programmes, based on successful skill acquisition rather than longevity, provide recognition for the significant contribution of the expert nurse to patient care. A flexible practice environment in which the expert is allowed to make exceptions to the rules in order to deliver better patient care is essential (Whitley 1992).

Expert nurses should be encouraged to attend educational programmes, not as a performance reward but rather as a recognized essential element for the advancement of their role and the advancement of nursing practice.

Similarly, strategies should be enacted that foster the development of the novice to become an expert oncology nurse. Whitley (1992) recommends that nurses who demonstrate the proficiency to become experts should be paired with a mentor. The mentor or clinical preceptor coordinates the novice's learning activities and functions as the primary role model and clinical resource. Mentors should not be in competition with the protégé (Cooley, Spatz & Yasko 1996) but should be confident enough in their own right to want the person being mentored to succeed them. Various mentors should be utilized throughout the development of the novice nurse. A satisfactory experience with a mentor can help develop the personal qualities and clinical expertise a novice oncology nurse needs to support individuals and families through a difficult experience (Johnson, Cohen & Hull 1994).

Lastly, membership of professional organizations and participation in institution-based committees can broaden professional horizons and present a new outlook on patient care for the developing expert cancer nurse (Whitley 1992).

Advanced practice

Debate is arising in Europe as well as North America over advanced practice in oncology nursing. The Advanced Practice Oncology Nurse, as defined by the Oncology Nursing Society (ONS), is prepared at a minimum of the master's degree in nursing, has direct and indirect clinical foci in the care of persons affected by cancer, and works in collaboration with nurse colleagues in practice, education, administration and research (ONS 1995, p. 45).* The ONS uses this term to designate the clinical nurse specialist (CNS) and nurse practitioner (NP) in oncology nursing and/or other master's-prepared nurses in education, administration or research. While both the CNS and NP roles evolved in response to social demand for affordable and accessible primary healthcare as well as to meet the demands of specialized care brought on through increasingly complex patient needs (Jacobs & Kreamer 1997), these two groups of expert nurses have traditionally carried out their roles in diversely different ways. Whereas the CNS role is more prevalent in acute care settings where the primary object of activity is the education and support of nursing staff, NPs are more often employed in ambulatory or home care settings, and activities focus on direct care of the patient and family (Page & Arena 1994).

In the United States, the roles of the CNS and NP are being merged in clinical settings as well as in graduate programmes of study. Current debate over this merger centres over the following issues. First, what is the type and scope of tasks and responsibilities these advanced nurses should assume, and is the assumption of these tasks economically driven? Justification of costs for a CNS, who is often not involved in direct patient care, is difficult. Similarly costly are physicians in training at a hospital. An advanced practice nurse could perform both roles at an economical advantage. Second, is this merger a step backward in that it abandons the struggle for nurse researchers and educators to provide the profession with theory-based nursing research to guide clinical practice in favour of the medical model (Page & Arena 1994)? The NP role is a more medically based model of nursing practice. The CNS has often been called the nurses' nurse. Proposed models for merging the two roles do not mention the new CNS role as modelling expert nursing care, and supporting and developing nursing personnel (Page & Arena 1994). Lastly, a crucial question arises from the CNS–NP debate which has little to do with role function: what is the contribution of advanced practice nurses to the quality of patient care (Jacobs & Kreamer 1997, Page & Arena 1994)?

The CNS and NP models of advanced practice in nursing have been instrumental in advancing the profession of nursing. Although their approach differs, these two types of specialists demonstrate the importance of experts in the care of designated groups of patients and how expert care affects patient outcome. In many institutions, these roles have already been merged. Page & Arena (1994) acknowledge that increased patient acuity, advances in technology and the arduous challenge to maintain quality in managed care environments all indicate a need to re-examine the role of advanced nurses. They caution, however, that the hasty merger of these two models of speciality care may have adverse consequences for both the profession of nursing and the quality of healthcare.

OUTLOOK FOR THE FUTURE

Cancer care knowledge for generalist nurses

The reality of the situation of cancer treatment in Europe is such that the majority of patients with cancer are not treated in cancer centres and/or university-affiliated

---

* Uniformly accepted definitions of the terms advanced practitioner and clinical nurse specialist do not currently exist in Europe. A panEuropean working group, supported by the European Network of Nursing Organizations (ENNO), was formed in 1998 to explore the feasibility of developing definitions and educational criteria for these roles.

hospitals. This situation is unlikely to change soon and, considering the increased incidence of cancer, it is also unlikely that all persons with cancer can and could be accommodated in cancer centres. This means that colleagues in general practice (practising in acute, home and ambulatory areas) need to enhance their knowledge of cancer care if patients are to receive optimal care. It is the responsibility of specialist nurses to disseminate their knowledge and experience and to provide consultative services to these colleagues in order to ensure that all persons with cancer in Europe obtain the same quality of nursing care.

Further direction of specialization

Specialty nursing groups in Europe are currently experiencing difficulty in receiving the recognition they deserve. For the professional nurse, this lack of recognition is frustrating and demoralizing. In Europe at a political level this lack of recognition has a profound effect on both monetary (i.e. salary) issues and on issues of status and power. EONS is working with other European specialist nursing groups to raise awareness of the significance of specialty nursing groups with appropriate EU legislative organizations. Individual nurses and national cancer nursing organizations must become proactive in strengthening the profile of cancer nurses at local, regional and national levels.

One question that will surely surface as a result of the further evolution of the specialty of cancer nursing is: should a qualifying process be developed in Europe to certify nurses who have already achieved the minimum credentials to practise as specialists? Certification processes usually take the form of a written examination based on specialty practice standards, and are issued by a nursing organization. Supporters of certification examinations contend that certification makes a difference to patients, employers, and to the individual nurse. For the patient, certification provides assurance the nurse has obtained the knowledge and skill that will enable him or her competently to provide specialized care (ONCC 1997). Certification signifies to the employer that a nurse has met or exceeded rigorous criteria for knowledge and experience, and is committed to the specialty. Preparation for the examination increases knowledge of cancer and cancer nursing practice. 'Attainment of the credential is a personal achievement that can boost self-esteem and increase self-confidence' (ONCC 1997). While successful certification allows the individual nurse to acquire distinction within a professional organization, recognition in terms of career advancement or increased earning potential remain administrative decisions to be determined by the employing institution (ONCC 1997). The question of whether other healthcare professionals will recognize the attainment of certified specialist knowledge and what certification represents is yet to be answered.

In 1997, EONS formed a working group to develop a procedure for the accreditation of continuing education courses for nurses in cancer care. The accreditation scheme was launched in 1999. Organizations and institutions that offer continuing education can submit courses for review and possible EONS accreditation. Work is ongoing on the development of a procedure for the accreditation of individual nurses. Certainly, the advantages of a standardized certification examination for the continued development of cancer nursing in Europe are numerous.

These issues are described in more detail in Chapter 5, or more information can be obtained from EONS.

Future roles of cancer nurses

Engelking (1994) predicts that there will be a resurgence in interest in the mind–body interrelationship in the next century. People will be more interested in self-care to prevent or shorten illness and improve quality of life (Engelking 1994).

Future goals of interventions, therefore, will be more concerned with disease prevention and helping persons to stay healthy in response to demand from the public for such services. Nurses could perform health examinations and physical assessments, provide health education and information on known cancer risks, perform diagnostic procedures and, with advanced education, provide genetic counselling to patients at risk of familial cancers (Young Summers & Chisholm 1997).

In addition to providing education related to prevention and psychosocial interventions to assist patients and families to learn to live with disease, opportunities will present themselves for nurses to become more independent of the medical establishment in terms of their practice. Legislation for such services is still lacking in some countries and it will be up to nurses to secure the necessary legal rights to practise independently. The provision of supportive care interventions to patients of all ages and at all phases of cancer as independent practitioners is a future role for advanced cancer nurse specialists. The elderly, men and children, traditionally underrepresented populations in terms of users of non-medical services, will be target groups for these interventions.

As the Internet and digital information become more prominent in everyday life, with it will come a deluge of information on cancer. The nurse's role in ongoing evaluation of cancer-related information available on the information highway will increase in importance, as will the nursing role as provider of such information.

Future opportunities for cancer nurses will be contingent on their ability to configure roles for themselves that allow for continued influence on the provision of healthcare (Young Summers & Chisholm 1997). It will become increasingly important for nurses to become politically astute, not only in terms of legislative measures that impact on practice, but also measures that affect funding for all types of cancer services. Nurses must, however, be prepared to go out and seize these opportunities and be able to justify the relevance of their role in cancer care.

Future sites of specialist practice

If current trends in the provision of healthcare services continue, it is safe to predict that the nurse of the future will provide care in a setting other than a hospital. Ambulatory care has proven to be less expensive and more efficient than treatment delivered in hospital, even when highly complex and technical procedures and treatments are administered (Young Summers & Chisholm 1977). It deserves mentioning that a rapidly growing area of future practice for specialist cancer nurses will be care of the elderly. Effective nursing management may be severely affected by the paucity of this information. The settings for care of the elderly may range from private homes to assisted living centres to elderly care institutions. Redmond & Aapro (1997) stress that the elderly often receive less than adequate cancer treatment on the basis of chronological age alone. Skilled specialists contribute to cost containment through recognition and intervention of complications that necessitate hospital admission and prudent intervention to avoid hospitalization. Young Summers & Chisholm (1997) note that some patients prefer treatment in ambulatory settings. Quality of life can be enhanced if patients are able to spend more time in their home environment.

CONCLUSION

Anticipated breakthroughs to find a cure for cancer have not yet materialized. While advances in the basic sciences have improved our understanding of the biology of cancer, most causes of cancer remain elusive. People will be affected by cancer for many years to come. These and other factors, including an increase in the sophistication of knowledge required to manage cancer symptoms, escalating healthcare costs, changing population demographics and advances in the profession of nursing, will continue to drive the demand for expert care.

The provision of the best possible cancer care intended to address the complex needs of patients and their families poses a daily challenge for cancer nursing specialists. This challenge is intensified in light of the changing economic structure of healthcare, which mandates providing more care in less time. Despite adverse conditions, cancer nurses are experts at caring for patients, and specialist cancer nurses are valuable resources for the continued provision of quality cancer care. Further study is needed to evaluate the cost effectiveness of their care. The future role of specialists and advanced practice nurses should not, however, be decided solely on economic criteria but rather on the impact of specialist care on the patient's outcome.

REFERENCES

Ash C R 1986 Cancer nursing in the year 2000. Cancer Nursing 9(1):A17

Benner P 1984 From novice to expert: excellence and power in clinical nursing practice. Addison-Wesley, Menlo Park, California

Boyle D M, Engelking C, Harvey C 1994 Taking command of the future: getting ready now for the 21st century. Oncology Nursing Forum 21(1):77–79

Caplan G 1970 The theory and practice of mental health consultation. Basic Books, New York

Cooley M E, Spatz D L, Yasko J M 1996 Role implications in cancer nursing. In: McCorkle R, Grant M, Frank-Stromborg, Baird S B (eds) Cancer nursing: a comprehensive textbook. W B Saunders, Philadelphia, ch 3, p 25

Corner J 1997 Beyond survival rates and side effects: cancer nursing as therapy. Cancer Nursing 20(1):3–11

Delleport W 1997 In memoriam: Robert Tiffany 1942–1993: introduction to the Robert Tiffany lecture. Cancer Nursing 20(1):1–2

Engelking C 1994 New approaches: innovations in cancer prevention, diagnosis, treatment, and support. Oncology Nursing Forum 21(1):62–71

Enghofer E 1997 Onkologie 2000 – Lehre, Forschung, Krankenversorgung: die zukunft der onkologie. Forum DKG 12:33–45

Esteves J, Kricker J F, Ferlay J, Parkin D M 1993 Facts and figures of cancer in the European community. Lyon: International Agency for Research on Cancer

European Oncology Nursing Society 1999 A core curriculum for a post-registration course in cancer nursing, 2nd edn. European Oncology Nursing Society, Brussels

Haberman M R, Germino B B, Maliski S, Stafford-Fox V, Rice K 1994 What makes oncology nursing special? Walking the road together. Oncology Nursing Forum 21(suppl 8):41–47

Hanneman S K 1996 Advancing nursing practice with a unit-based clinical expert. Image: Journal of Nursing Scholarship 28(4):331–337

Jacobs L H, Kreamer K M 1997 The oncology clinical nurse specialist in a post master's nurse practitioner program: a personal and professional journey. Oncology Nursing Forum 24(8):1387–1392

Johnson L R, Cohen M Z, Hull M M 1994 Cultivating expertise in oncology nursing: methods, mentors, and memories. Oncology Nursing Forum 21(suppl 8):27–34

Landis S H, Murray T, Bolden S, Wingo P A 1998 Cancer statistics, 1998. CA: A Cancer Journal for Clinicians 48(1):6–29

McCorkle R, Grant M, Frank-Stromborg M, Baird S B 1996 Cancer nursing as a specialty. In: McCorkle R, Grant M, Frank-Stromborg M, Baird S B (eds) Cancer nursing: a comprehensive textbook. W B Saunders, Philadelphia, ch 1, p 1

Oncology Nursing Certification Corporation 1997 Certification makes a difference brochure. Oncology Nursing Press, Pittsburgh

Oncology Nursing Society 1995 Position statement on advanced practice nursing in oncology nursing. Oncology Nursing Forum 22(suppl 8):45

Page N E, Arena D 1994 Rethinking the merger of the clinical nurse specialist and the nurse practitioner. Image: Journal of Nursing Scholarship 26:315–318

Redmond K, Aapro M S (eds) 1997 Cancer in the elderly: a nursing and medical perspective. Elsevier Science, Amsterdam

Stetz K, Haberman M R, Holcombe J, Jones L 1995 1994 ONS research priorities survey. Oncology Nursing Forum 22(5):785–789

Watson P G 1996 Rehabilitation services. In: McCorkle R, Grant M, Frank-Stromborg M, Baird S B (eds) Cancer nursing: a comprehensive textbook. W B Saunders, Philadelphia, ch 75, p 1300

Whitley M J 1992 Characteristics of the expert oncology nurse. Oncology Nursing Forum 19(8):1242–1246

Wright S 1992 Modelling excellence: the role of the consultant nurse. In: Butterworth T, Fungier S (eds) Clinical supervision and mentorship in nursing. Chapman and Hall, London, ch 15, p 203

Yarbro C H 1996 The history of cancer nursing. In: McCorkle R, Grant M, Frank-Stromborg M, Baird S B (eds) Cancer nursing: a comprehensive textbook. W B Saunders, Philadelphia, ch 2, p 12

Yasko J M 1991 Role implementation in cancer nursing. In: Baird S B, McCorkle R, Grant M (eds) Cancer nursing: a comprehensive textbook. W B Saunders, Philadelphia, ch 3, p 21

Young Summers B L, Chisholm L M 1997 Opportunities and challenges for oncology nursing in ambulatory cancer care. Oncology Nursing Updates 4(1):1–14

The practice base of cancer nursing

Karin Magnusson   Lorraine Robinson

CHAPTER 2

THE ESSENCE OF CANCER NURSING

In a scientific discipline, in this case cancer nursing, practice is derived from the knowledge base of the discipline. Smith (1994) considers that the distinctiveness of our practice – what we offer as nurses – emerges from the distinctiveness of our knowledge. Cody & Mitchell (1992) state that 'if nursing practice is the performing art of the science of nursing, then practice is guided by nursing theory and cannot be considered separately from it' (p. 52). In this context the concept of nursing theory refers specifically to 'a distinct and well-articulated system of concepts and propositions rooted explicitly in a philosophy of nursing and intended solely to guide nursing practice and research' (Cody 1994, p. 144). According to Dorsett (1993) nursing, as a caring science, is based on a theoretical foundation for practice, continuously tested, refined and verified by research, and a clearly articulated set of principles guiding that practice. Central to the concept of quality of care is a set of standards that exists to guide practice by operationalizing its essence.

Cody (1994) states that nursing will achieve parity with other scholarly disciplines when nurses everywhere are guided in their practice by a theory base specific to nursing. Cody interprets nursing theory-guided practice to be practice that is based on theory and is specific to the discipline of nursing, explicitly rooted in the philosophy of nursing, and intended solely to guide nursing practice and research. Nursing theory can facilitate the development of practice methods or traditions. According to Morse & Werner (1988), the diagnosis and treatment of human responses to actual or potential health problems can be linked effectively to nursing theory, especially to one concerned with sustenance of life and health, recovery from illness and coping with its effects.

Therefore, there should also be a coherent connection between practice and research. Leininger (1981) states that the theory–research–practice linkage: (a) provides a basis for thinking and decision-making, (b) provides a 'holistic' nursing perspective, (c) promotes the use of substantive knowledge in practice, (d) stimulates the intellectual and humanistic aspects of nursing, thus combating routinization of care, and (e) provides a common language which facilitates communication and promotes common goals.

In the case of cancer nursing, common goals are to improve health, well-being and quality of life, and to evaluate nursing care incorporating qualitative measures as described by those receiving care. Clinical competence, accessibility, supportive intervention, ability to communicate, a nonjudgemental attitude and the nurse's ability to meet patients' distress with empathy are important factors in the sphere of cancer nursing practice. In these areas of practice it is vital constantly to subject both the research evidence and theoretical constructs to critical appraisal.

Quality of life, for example, is an appropriate outcome measure for evaluating the impact of cancer nursing care (Padilla & Grant 1985) given that many nursing activities impact on the patient's quality of life (Glaus 1993). Nursing interventions or care delivered within the framework of the nursing process may directly or indirectly impact on quality of life. For example, in a study by Padilla & Grant

(1985) nurse availability and patient confidence in nurses were significantly correlated with patient well-being. According to Cella (1993), nursing has always played a central role in determining that quality of life be considered an important outcome when evaluating the efficacy of treatment and care. This is evidenced by interest in, and commitment to, managing disease symptoms and treatment side-effects, offering family-centred care and focusing on the psychosocial impact of the cancer experience.

A survey by Rieker, Clarke & Fogelberg (1992) investigated how both 'quality of life' and 'quality of care' were perceived by patients, treated with biological therapy, and their relatives. The results showed that four components were significant in both patients' and family members' assessment of quality of care: availability of support services, adequate symptom control, communication with the medical team, and adequate information about how medical care was proceeding. However, Glaus (1993) considers that quality of life and quality of care are interrelated. According to Glaus, 'the perception of the quality of care is very influenced by ways of coping: feelings of anger and hostility, due to disease progression, often are directed against treatment methods and even against care givers' (p. 121). As nurses, we respect the beliefs and values of patients with cancer when they choose how to live and how to die. The cancer nurse has an important role as the patient's advocate in any healthcare system. We must meet patients' needs with the care we provide and continually evaluate that care in the light of changing healthcare needs, developments in cancer care treatment and delivery, and advances in nursing practice.

The concept of care

Caring has emerged as a central concept for nursing, and has even been described by Leininger (1988) as the essence of nursing and a central dominant feature. If nursing is about care, and hence care is at the core of cancer nursing, what then is care? There is no universal definition of care, but it has been identified as the essence and unifying domain for the body of knowledge in nursing (Leininger 1981). Clarke & Wheeler (1992) argue that, to date, the literature offers two dimensions of caring: a definitional approach (Leininger 1981, Watson 1979) and an approach focusing on meaning and the intuitive values of caring (Benner & Wrubel 1989, Forrest 1989). Care is an overall concept and is founded on ethical choices and philosophical values based on a humanistic perspective (Watson 1985). Watson (1985) states that, through caring, the nurse helps another human being to gain self-knowledge, self-control and self healing, and that in the caring process both the patient and the nurse have the possibility to grow. She defines caring as a process that helps a person to attain or maintain health or a peaceful death (Watson 1979). Caring behaviour in nursing is manifest through the attributes of compassion, competence, confidence, conscience and commitment (Roach 1987).

However, several care researchers are critical about the use of the term care as a central concept in nursing. For example, Lützén & Barbosa da Silva (1995) consider that care as the central concept of nursing can create ethical problems, and can be confused with notions of paternalism and 'knowing what is best' for the patient.

The importance of sensitive and efficient cancer care that gives priority to caring and not only curing in a manner that is meaningful to the patient has been emphasized in the literature (Halldórsdóttir & Hamrin 1997). Padilla & Grant (1985) assert that in caring for the person with cancer 'the nurse's role is frequently one of helping the patient to manage the side effects of therapy and to adjust to the permanent changes in body image, function and appearance'

(p. 45). They also support the notion that the quality of the patient's survival may be 'associated not only with the inherent personal strength of the patient, but also with how well the nurse is able to help the patient with needed changes and adjustments' (p. 45). Therefore, caring establishes itself as a concept central to the everyday practice of cancer nursing with a potential impact on the course and quality of the patient's and family's experience. The challenge is to demonstrate this facet of cancer nursing practice through research and in terms of specific outcome measures.

Notion of holism

Cancer nursing practice, it can be argued, is also based on the notion of holism. Holism implies the integration of parts to achieve harmony (Griffin 1993). From a holistic perspective, consideration is given to instant and continuous interaction between the individual, his or her environment and health. According to Gaut (1993), a caring, holistic perspective involves seeking a pattern rather than cause and effect. This approach to care requires the professional carer to see pain and disease not as something evil in itself but as a source of information about the conflict and imbalance the person experiences and responds to (Gaut 1993).

Holism is exemplified in the acknowledgment and treatment of the person with cancer as a being with biological, psychological, spiritual and social needs. This includes the acceptance of cancer as a 'family disease' (Welch-McCaffrey 1983). One way to work holistically is to allow the patient to keep his or her personality in the care situation. Hospice care is an example of a holistic approach where the care focuses on physical, psychological, social and spiritual needs; and includes the family as well as the patient (Athlin et al 1993). It is perhaps easy for the discipline to associate itself with holism; the more difficult task is to make the philosophy of holism a reality in cancer nursing practice. This chapter will focus largely on the nature of cancer nursing practice and thereby consider the very essence of the specialty. In the following sections the development and expansion of cancer nursing will be explored. Central to many of these developments is a commonly held belief that providing a more holistic service for persons with cancer has been at the heart of innovations in care. As yet, we have not delineated as a discipline whether these ideas are mere rhetoric or whether in reality the experience of care for the person with cancer is a holistic one.

DEVELOPMENT OF A NURSING SPECIALTY

It is argued that caring and holism are concepts that reflect the essence of cancer nursing and it is therefore important to consider the development of cancer nursing as a nursing specialty. Lützén & Barbosa da Silva (1995) suggest that there are at least two possible explanations for the birth of a new science and the processes that stimulate its growth. The new science may either appear in response to unmet concrete needs in the society or evolve from a parent discipline in which accepted theories are insufficient to explain new problems. The foundation stone for the nursing discipline was laid in the Nightingale era, when nursing leaders argued that nursing knowledge and practice were different from medicine (Cameron-Traub 1991). Today the differentiation between nursing and medicine is the primary or main focus, which for nursing is interpersonal interactions and for medicine is technological intervention (Chinn & Jacobs 1987).

In response to changes in nursing generally, biomedical advances and cultural and social expectations of healthcare, cancer nursing has evolved and continues to develop. For example, historically, it was the role of the research nurse to assist in clinical trials of cancer treatments that involved cancer nursing (Corner 1997).

Corner (1997) considers that the value of skilled nursing in administering cytotoxic therapies and supporting patients was recognized at this time. The 1970s was a time of extension and expansion of the role and function of the nurse in cancer care and of the growth of educational programmes designed to prepare nurses to meet these challenging demands (Tiffany 1987).

Therefore, the range and scope of practice of cancer nursing is continually evolving. A patient with cancer may pass through several phases in the course of the disease (e.g. screening, the prediagnostic phase, diagnosis, treatment, remission, recurrence, and death and dying). Each of these phases constitutes an important step in the patient's situation (Benner & Wrubel 1989). Cancer nursing addresses all stages of the cancer experience and the varied and changing needs for information, symptom control and supportive care. Alongside taking care of the patient's physical, emotional and social needs, the nurse must, when it is needed, be technically skilled and, for example, be able to prepare and administer cytotoxics safely and effectively.

Expansion of the nurse's role in cancer nursing practice

There has been a rapid expansion to the traditional role of the nurse and development of new roles for nurses, for example the clinical nurse specialists (CNSs), nurse practitioners and nurses as primary healthcare workers. The CNS is responsible for direct care of selected patients, consultation with nurse specialists in different clinical areas and with nurses in general practice, and collaboration in planning care for individuals or groups of patients (American Nurses Association 1985). The role of the oncology clinical nurse specialist (OCNS) is described by Siehl (1982) as to assist nurses and other health professionals to find a balance between what is and what ought to be. According to Welch-McCaffrey (1986), it is important for each nursing specialty to identify the practice elements that are appropriate for consultation by the CNS. Welch-McCaffrey (1986) suggests that, in cancer nursing, the OCNS should be expert in, and a resource person for, problems associated with: (a) physical status management, (b) patient and family education, (c) psychosocial support, and (d) resource facilitation.

Alongside the development of the OCNS, the nurse can play a leading part in the team during screening for cancer diseases such as malignant melanoma, breast cancer and cancer of the cervix. The need for genetic counselling is also increasing as the work of elucidating the importance of genetic mutations as a cause of cancer advances (Kelly 1992). The potential rising need for genetic counselling means that an increasing number of nurses are trained as genetic counsellors. With appropriate education and training, the nurse can play a prominent part in the investigative work, the counselling process and the psychosocial management in this area of practice.

As the potential scope of cancer nursing practice increases in the prediagnosis phase, cancer nursing has also begun to establish a role in rehabilitation of persons with cancer. Rehabilitative nursing is an integral part of all phases of patient-centred care. The role of the nurse in addressing rehabilitation issues for persons with cancer is one of teaching, counselling and coordination (Anderson 1989). Anderson (1989) also states that nurses have made significant contributions to educational programmes available to persons with cancer and their families. They have developed site-specific support programmes, as well as programmes that identify and support positive coping behaviours for the person with cancer.

Different kinds of nurse-led clinics are becoming increasingly common. New treatment regimens require re-examination of old assumptions about patient needs and the delivery of care. A nurse-led clinic is one possible solution in meeting the ongoing needs of patients during the treatment phase of their illness experience.

Cancer nursing care in a radiotherapy department may involve offering help with the management of side-effects, psychosexual care, facilitating coping and patient education, for example (Wengstrom & Haggmark 1998).

In some healthcare settings the cancer nurse has a pivotal role in the multi-professional team. There are various areas where teamwork could be strengthened and there are opportunities to share expertise and experience within the wider team (Carson et al 1997). The wider team in cancer care can involve personnel other than nurses, such as doctors, physiotherapists, dietitians, occupational thera-pists, social workers, psychologists, etc. Practising cancer nurses have a key role to play in the multiprofessional team and the development of collaborative working within cancer care.

Delivery systems and continuity for cancer care

Cancer care is delivered in a wide range of healthcare settings, for example in hospitals (e.g. specialist units, day-care clinics, general wards), community care, primary healthcare, home care and in hospices. The role of the nurse may be very different in different settings and the focus of interaction is influenced by that con-text of care. However, whatever the setting, continuity of care is important. This is because continuity of care implies a standard in which there is planned coordina-tion of care that results in an improved outcome for the patient, irrespective of the care setting or provider (Ferrell & O'Neil-Page 1993). One way to achieve continu-ity is to adopt the primary nursing model, an organizational model of nursing care, which implies that a nurse acts as a coordinator for all aspects of the person's care (Macguire 1989).

Pyles & Stern (1983) consider that the nurse's intuition is an important tool in the provision of care. Clinical observation and assessment were proved in their study to be related to what is sometimes called 'clinical decision processes'. They state that nurses learn how to observe, what to observe and how to draw conclu-sions from their observations, and that this knowledge is fundamental to the diag-nostic process. Pyles & Stern (1983) also argue that nurses have the ability to detect signs at an early stage as they are constantly in the clinical area and see the patient under everyday conditions. Continuity of care, seen by all practitioners as a central component in cancer nursing practice, is therefore important in creating the oppor-tunity for nurses to establish realistic and credible nursing diagnoses.

The maintenance of continuity of care has been brought sharply into focus because in recent years there have been changes in the focus of care for the increas-ing number of patients. This includes increased emphasis on outpatient and com-munity care and patient informed choice (Smith & Richardson 1996). This is due, among other things, to the increasing costs of inpatient treatment, policy direc-tives, demands from patients themselves (Smith & Richardson 1996) and advances in biomedical technology (Reville & Almadrones 1989). For example, in the area of outpatient chemotherapy, important factors that influence the delivery of care and continuity include the use of catheters and ports, as well as implantable and exter-nal pumps for continuous infusions and use of oral chemotherapy when possible (Yasko & Rust 1989).

The nurse engaged in cancer care must consider the chain of care and remember that for many patients a single treatment session may constitute a link in a long chain of measures, for instance between outpatient and inpatient care. It can be argued that cancer nurses can provide a vital link in promoting continuity of care through interprofessional communication, documentation, dialogue with the patient and family, facilitating access to information, financial, social, voluntary and charity sector resources, and adopting a person-centred rather that disease-centred approach to care.

Nursing intervention

Corner (1997) has discussed the phrase 'nursing as therapy', a term used by McMahon & Pearson (1991). Corner (1997) believes that there is clear evidence of the therapeutic effects of cancer nursing interventions from a series of meta-analyses. According to Meutzel's model, the core of therapeutic nursing practice is partnership, intimacy and reciprocity (Muetzel 1988). Through recourse to the literature Corner (1997) discovered two further elements of therapeutic nursing: 'the use of reflection and evaluation of experience as an integral and ongoing process of everyday practice and *presence* in the psychotherapeutic sense of *being there* and *being with* clients' (p. 6). These further elements are based on the work of Powell (1991) and Ersser (1991) respectively. Through this, nurses deliver therapeutic care by manipulating the environment, teaching, providing comfort, adopting complementary health practices and utilizing physical interventions (Corner 1997).

Nursing interventions in connection with cancer are largely a question of cooperation and communication between the nurse and patient. Orem (1985) emphasizes the importance of the relationship between patient and nurse, its quality, and the need for the nurse to employ both her professional know-how and communication skills in dealing with patients. Orem also contends that the structure of care depends on actions that are thoroughly considered, selected and carried out by nurses to help individuals or groups to maintain or alter conditions in themselves or their surroundings. This can be achieved by self-care under the nurse's supervision or by the nurse when a person's possibilities are limited owing to impaired health.

A very important part of cancer nursing is control of symptoms, related to cancer and/or its treatment, which have a potential or actual impact on the patient's quality of life. The outcome of poorly controlled symptoms, besides impaired quality of life, may be despair, decreased energy, carer burden, compromised survivorship and complicated bereavement (Hogan 1997). Identification of patients who need supportive interventions requires repeated interactions with the patient and family, and involves assessing mental and physical reaction to treatment, inquiring about 'areas of concern' and inviting patients to talk over quality-of-life issues (Bolund 1990). Goodman (1989) states that 'the nurse's assessment of a patient's response to therapy and assistance in preventing or managing even the most common side effect can make the difference in the patient's overall response to cancer treatment' (p. 29). Hogan (1997) points out that there are some barriers to effective symptom control, such as poor communication, professional rivalry, inadequate knowledge, cost, the 'we have always done it this way' syndrome, inadequate administrative support and 'old wives' tales'. Despite this, we can today, if we apply the knowledge available, often help the patient with control of many symptoms (e.g. fatigue, diarrhoea, nausea and vomiting, body image, mucositis and pain).

Several sources of evidence suggest that psychosocial factors play a role in the patient's experience of treatment toxicity, for example that pharmacological effects do not explain the variable frequency and severity of a number of adverse reactions. The phenomenon of pretreatment nausea, for instance, is explained as a conditioned psychological response and cross-cultural variation exists, substantiating psychosocial influence (Cassileth, Lusk & Bodenheimer 1985). Cassileth's study of patients about to receive chemotherapy for the first time indicates a lack of accord between patients' expectations about side-effects and their actual experience.

An important task for the cancer nurse in relation to symptom management is therefore to offer the person with cancer a realistic view of treatment or intervention, and to provide appropriate information relating to self-care strategies. Teaching about self-care is an attempt to provide a model of care that equips individuals with strategies to manage their care, symptoms or treatment experience, or throughout a lifetime if appropriate (O'Malley, Loveridge & Cummings 1989). Orem (1985) has developed a model that is based on the premise that all persons require self-care in order to maintain health and life. According to Orem's model of nursing, a self-care deficit exists when an individual's self-care agency is inadequate to meet the therapeutic self-care demands, and this condition signals the need for nursing service (Fernsler 1986). Facilitating self-care in patients with cancer is essential to providing quality nursing care and the nurse's responsibility for direct patient care now includes educating the patient toward self-care (Dodd 1982). According to Stromberg (1986), teaching self-care may encourage persons with cancer to increase their sense of self-control and lessen the feelings of helplessness that often accompany cancer and its treatment.

Communication and cancer nursing

Communication is a central concept in cancer nursing. There is growing research evidence of the high informational needs of patients with cancer (e.g. Derdiarian 1987a,b, Grahn & Johnson 1990). This appears to be irrespective of cancer type, ethnicity or other demographic characteristics (Graydon et al 1997), although there is conflicting evidence of the informational needs of patients related to stage of disease. Some authors suggest that those with early disease have greater information needs than those with advanced disease (e.g. Brandt 1991), whereas others contend that those surviving cancer or facing recurrence and advanced disease have an equally high but different need for information (e.g. Mahon 1991, Pelusi 1997, Robinson 1994).

The cancer experience involves a number of complex communication-related issues for patients, their families and healthcare professionals, including: maintaining a sense of control, seeking information, disclosing feelings and searching for meaning (Northouse & Northouse 1987). Loss of control refers to a person's perceived ability to make choices that will affect events in their lives (Northouse & Northouse 1987). Blumberg, Flaherty & Lewis (1980) posit that loss of control also brings with it a sense of dependence, lack of autonomy and feelings of vulnerability. Gaining a sense of control may be difficult for patients associated with the cause, diagnosis, treatment and prognosis of cancer (e.g. Cohn 1982, Peters-Golden 1982). Seeking information is closely related to a person's need to maintain control (e.g. Felton & Revenson 1984, Mishel et al 1984) and is perceived as beneficial as it offers a framework for clarifying life-threatening events (Northouse & Northouse 1987).

Receiving the right amount and type of information is important for individuals with cancer; a cancer diagnosis is still regarded with more fear than other diagnoses, instilling feelings of shock, grief, uncertainty and loss of control (Northouse & Northouse 1987). In diagnoses where a choice of treatment may exist, for example breast cancer, it is of particular importance that the nurse provides adequate information (Luker et al 1995). Luker and colleagues (1995) found in their study that women with newly diagnosed breast cancer had a 'top three information need', namely likelihood of cure, spread of disease and treatment options. They contend that this information provision may fall within the scope of practice of the specialist breast care nurse. The nurse could also act as a facilitator, enabling patients to gain access to important information by making medical colleagues aware of their information needs.

Self-disclosure, it has been contended, is closely related to healthy adjustment (Jourard 1971). Silver & Wortman (1980) outline that disclosing feelings assists patients with cancer in receiving feedback, facilitates problem-solving and allows ventilation of feelings. Patients with cancer can, however, be inhibited in disclosing their feelings. Mitchell & Glicksman (1977), for example, found that most of the 50 patients undergoing radiotherapy in their study were afraid to share their feelings with the physician as they considered them to be too busy. The research, although minimal, does indicate the benefits for patients of disclosing their feelings. During the experience of cancer people are sometimes faced with a sense of confusion over the meaning of their lives (Northouse & Northouse 1987). The intervention study carried out by Spiegel, Bloom & Yalom (1981), which examined the psychological benefit of support groups for individuals with metastatic breast cancer, highlighted that 'supportive, direct confrontation with life-and-death issues would result in a sense of mastery rather than demoralisation' (Northouse & Northouse 1987, p. 27).

The subject of cancer is an emotionally charged area and nurses often feel limited in their ability to communicate in an effective way (Wilkinson 1991). Nurses often use simple, everyday, informal language. According to Bourhis, Roth & MacQueen (1989), this often replaces medical language, making it easier to communicate with patients and their families. For seriously ill patients, a good relationship with the nurse may be particularly important. Patients who have confidence in their nurse may be glad to allow him or her to act as their advocate and speak on their behalf if and when they are unable to plead their own case. Conversation is also a means of establishing or strengthening the relationship between patient and nurse, and of giving emotional support. In certain cases, body language, alone or in combination with a verbal message, may also be a means of communication for the patient.

STRESS AND CANCER NURSING PRACTICE

As the next millennium approaches, we have taken the opportunity to look at the range, scope and potential of cancer nursing practice. We have argued that practice is the essence of cancer nursing and discussed the values that are central to the specialty and the delivery of individualized, sensitive and contemporary cancer nursing care. However, it is essential to also examine what Larson (1992) describes as the challenge of caring. Cancer nurses do not work in isolation from the experiences of the individuals and families for whom they care, or their healthcare colleagues. Nor are they unaware of the local, national, cultural and political context that impinges on the views of cancer nursing and affects, directly and indirectly, its resourcing.

Today, there is a burgeoning literature focused on stress and burnout for the helping professions and it is generally acknowledged that nursing is a stressful occupation. However, in the quest to demonstrate which areas of nursing are most stressful, or experience the highest levels of burnout, a key point, fundamental to cancer nursing practice, has often been excluded from the debate and has only recently begun to be addressed in detail. That is the intimate relationship between caring and stress.

Despite its prevalence in everyday life, stress appears to have eluded clarity and consensus concerning a definition. The early models were influenced by the two major views of stress. These are the classic formulations, associated with the work of Selye (1956), which identify the physiological and endocrinological processes, and the interactionist view propounded by the work of Lazarus (Lazarus 1966, Lazarus & Folkman 1984). Latterly Benner & Wrubel (1989) have linked the concepts of stress and caring. Caring in their phenomenological perspective means 'that persons, events, projects and things matter to people' (p. 1). Caring therefore establishes what is stressful. Benner & Wrubel (1989) state 'we do not view stress as a state that can always be avoided or even one that must always be "cured". Rather, stress is the inevitable result of living in a world where things matter to one' (p. 61). If cancer nursing holds caring as a central component of practice and cares about the experience of the patient, family and colleagues, then we will experience stress. Therefore, it is vital to understand the nature of this relationship in order to support the work of the nurse and his or her emotional well-being.

Within the sphere of cancer nursing it has been contended that most cancer nurses feel a strong sense of purpose in their work (Larson 1992). The literature and empirical research offer a number of explanations and perspectives on the challenges that existed for cancer nurses in relation to caring in the later part of the twentieth century. These will be explored in relation to the emotional labour of cancer nursing and issues of occupational stress and burnout.

Emotional labour of cancer nursing

Whether one views the experiences of cancer nurses as swinging from drama to tragedy and back, or simply as a rewarding and sometimes difficult job, there are issues about the emotional work that accompanies the day-to-day reality of being a cancer nurse that are worthy of exploration. These include: the relationships cancer nurses form with patients and their families; the intimacy and involvement this brings; working with the person with cancer who is facing a life-threatening and sometimes chronic disease; and caring for the dying patient with cancer and their family.

Caring, like stress, has been explored from several viewpoints. While caring is a component of the patient and family experience, it is also a key feature of the practice of cancer care from the perspective of the nurse. If it is argued that the very essence of cancer nursing is built on a caring relationship with the person with cancer, then it follows that the process of caring will have an impact, positive or otherwise, on the nurse. Researchers have attempted to understand the meaning of cancer nursing and its concomitant emotional labour through examination of communication issues, the interpersonal relationship between the nurse and patient, exploration of boundaries, intimacy and involvement with the patient with cancer and their family, and caring for the dying patient with cancer.

First, communicating with a person with cancer is generally accepted as a vital and influential aspect of nursing care (Faulkner & Maguire 1994, Macleod Clark 1982, Wilkinson 1991). However, cancer nurses' abilities to meet the communication needs of their client group have been questioned. While the informational needs of patients with cancer continue to be delineated through research (e.g. Graydon et al 1997, Hooker 1997, Luker et al 1995, 1996), communication research seems still to suggest that cancer nurses often fail to meet their potential contribution to the communication needs of patients with cancer.

Wilkinson (1991), for example, explored factors that influence how nurses communicate with patients with cancer. Predictors of facilitating verbal behaviour in interactions with patients included place of work, finding the delivery of poor care a major stressor, support from managers, postbasic education in cancer nursing, and nurses' own feelings about communicating with patients with cancer, and hobbies outside nursing. Similarly, predictors of blocking verbal behaviours included place of work, religion, self-awareness and nurses' own fear of death. Interestingly, nurses with the highest level of blocking behaviour had the lowest level of anxiety (measured with the State Trait Anxiety Inventory; Spielberger, Gorsch & Lushene 1983) after completing the most difficult nursing history. As with all research studies, Wilkinson's work is open to scrutiny (e.g. her oversimplification of nurses into facilitators or blockers), but the study does raise some interesting points. As Wilkinson (1991) concludes, effective communication does not depend entirely on the acquisition of communication skills. It is contended that the process and context of the communication need to be explored as well as the skills utilized. The gamut of factors identified by Wilkinson (1991) and others that are involved in the process of communication with individuals with cancer and their families leads us to consider the day-to-day stress of matching or feeling equipped with the appropriate interpersonal skill, responses to address the informational needs or emotional responses of the client and family, and the complex processes of interprofessional cancer care communication. However, it also compels us to examine the relationship that cancer nurses form with clients, patients and family members.

From our own reflections and personal experiences of cancer nursing, and our observations of colleagues, we know that the majority of cancer nurses form special and unique relationships with individuals and their families. Artinian (1995) explored the process of developing special relationships with patients with cancer. This study utilized open-ended interviews to explore the difference between the neutral relationships that nurses had with some patients and the special relationships they had with others. The researcher did not predefine special relationship for the participant; rather, this emerged from the nurse's own description. This paper offers insight into why cancer nurses risk involvement with patients and why they resist involvement with other patients. Artinian (1995) suggests that cancer nurses' attitudes about caring for people with cancer, the support available to them and previous experience of unresolved grief influence decisions related to risking emotional involvement. This small-scale study provides some interesting insights. It was suggested that the vulnerability of patients and the challenge posed for nursing care was an issue in selecting to pursue a more intimate relationship. The consequences of such an intimate relationship seemed to include acceptance of the sadness and physical responses that accompany grief but also the potential for unresolved grief.

Little has been written about the grief experience of cancer nurses. Stowers (1983) believes that nurses are seldom able to share the grief experienced when a person dies. Larson (1992) describes cancer nurses as 'working downstream', which is often frustrating and exhausting. This downstream work is not the entirety of cancer nursing practice but can account for a significant proportion of the work of some cancer nurses. Felstein & Gemma (1995) studied the grief of oncology nurses over a 1-year period, following 50 nurses (termed stayers and leavers). They argued that cancer nurses' involvement with seriously ill patients can generate emotional stress. We would concur with their premise that few nurses receive explicit practical preparation to assist them with the emotional component of caring for the person dying as a result of cancer. The researchers were unable to determine whether nurses who left oncology or transferred to another area of practice did so because of chronic compounded or unresolved grief. However, 38% of the sample did not answer the question related to professional grief, and a higher number of deaths were experienced by those that stayed in the oncology area. While conjecture is difficult, it does raise an important question about why cancer nurses were not able to answer a personal question about professional grief. Confrontations with death are not unusual for a cancer nurse. Felstein & Gemma (1995) posit that, although nurses' exposure to death and dying is a source of anxiety, 'there is often a covert institutional message as well as peer pressure not to dwell on the loss' (p. 229).

Conversely, more recent research again focuses on the reciprocity in relationships between cancer nurses and dying patients. Rittman et al (1997) report in their phenomenological study of nurses caring for patients dying as a result of cancer that nurses were committed to participating in the experience and developing meaningful relationships with patients and their families. From the analysis of in-depth interviews with six nurses, five themes emerged: (1) knowing the patient and their stage of illness, (2) preserving hope, (3) easing the struggle and promoting a peaceful death, (4) providing privacy, and (5) responding to spiritual aspects of the experience for both the nurse and the patient. What can be learned from a study such as this is that, in engaging in activities that many would regard as the cornerstone of cancer nursing, at any stage of the cancer experience nurses set up what is important to them in their relationships with patients with cancer, what matters, and thus what is found to be both rewarding and stressful. Separating, within the caring encounter, what is sustaining for the cancer nurse and what is stressful may be a moot point. Personal reflection and focused research will help us to establish the 'what is' aspect of cancer nursing practice and so potentially help us to be more specific about the how, why and when we support cancer nurses in the stressful milieu of cancer nursing practice. This is an alternative approach to endeavouring to separate stressful from non-stressful aspects of cancer nursing work.

This brings us to consider one of the challenges of caring identified specifically by Larson (1992), that of empathy. Larson (1992) describes empathy as 'a double-edged sword; it is simultaneously your greatest asset and a point of vulnerability' (p. 857). The challenge, therefore, is to find a way to be emotionally involved as a caregiver without burning out. Larson (1992) describes the work of Stotland and colleagues (1978), who found that new nurses who scored the highest on empathy scores became distressed when in the rooms of dying patients and were the first to leave. Support and advice on how to relate to the patients changed this scenario. Therefore, meeting the challenge is a complex task and requires support from colleagues, as well as individual inner resources. It can be difficult to be a self-sustaining cancer nurse in the current climate of healthcare across and within Europe because of resources, staff shortages and the expectations of the general public and professional colleagues. It is also important to note that the changing roles and boundaries of cancer nursing practice can also be conceived as both a source of stress and a potential reward. Instead, the task seems to lie in providing a supportive working environment that equips cancer nurses to provide competent, sensitive and contemporary cancer care in an ever-changing social, economic and political world. Perhaps what the previous discussion indicates is that, because of the emotional labour of cancer nursing and its commitment to the care of individuals and their families, the resource lies within the specialty itself to support ourselves and one another as cancer nurses. This will be discussed further in the latter part of the chapter when we examine the potential and scope for clinical supervision as a supportive strategy for cancer nursing practice.

Occupational stress and burnout in cancer nursing

So far we have examined what some may call 'internal factors' in relation to the emotional labour and stress of cancer nursing, that is, the relationships we form with patients with cancer, their families and friends, cancer nursing colleagues and other healthcare professionals, and also the consequences of dealing with these relationships and the needs and experiences during the cancer experience. It has been debated, in early reports, whether cancer nurses are at particular risk of developing 'burnout' because of their ongoing exposure to the distress cancer can create (McElroy 1982, Newlin & Wellisch 1978, Yano 1977).

A decade ago Delvaux et al (1988) commented that the literature relating to healthcare professionals dealing with the stress of cancer care was in its infancy. And two decades ago Oberst (1978) surveyed oncology nurses in the United States and determined that finding ways to prevent burnout was among the highest research priorities for practice-based cancer nurses. Presently similar points could be made. It is generally accepted that healthcare professionals are prime targets for occupational stress because, as Ogle (1983) suggests, 'their everyday work situations are associated with crisis, rapid decision making and fast-paced schedules' (p. 31). However, more recently research reports have disagreed about whether, in fact, cancer nurses are at any more risk of developing burnout than nurses working in other settings.

Research has addressed the stressors associated with cancer nursing and evaluated burnout amongst oncology nurses. The work of Maslach has been influential in developing assessment scales for measuring burnout (Maslach 1976, Maslach & Pines 1977). The Maslach Burnout Inventory utilizes measures to examine emotional exhaustion, depersonalization and personal accomplishment. Burnout is a syndrome described as emotional exhaustion (Jenkins & Ostchega 1986), although the effects can be demonstrated physically (e.g. fatigue, physical exhaustion, depression, sleeplessness), cognitively (e.g. impaired decision-making, inflexibility, cynicism) and psychologically (e.g. shift in attitudes to patients, anger, withdrawal, alteration in self-image) (Ogle 1983). The syndrome has been described as a critical issue for healthcare (Bram & Kratz 1989), and Muldary (1983) defines it as a 'highly variable complex of signs, symptoms and manifestations' (p. 43).

An example of such research is that of van Sevellen and Leake (1993), who examined burnout among hospital nurses working on AIDS units, special care units, oncology special care units, medical intensive care units and general medical units. They determined from a sample of 237 nurses from 18 units in seven hospitals that there was no significant difference in burnout scores across units. Nurses working in cancer care did not seem to experience more burnout than other clinically based nurses. This supported previous research by Jenkins & Ostchega (1986) whose study set out to determine whether cancer nurses experienced burnout and to what degree. The Staff Burnout Scale for Health Care Professionals (Jones 1980) demonstrated that cancer nurses did experience 'some degree of burnout' (Jenkins & Ostchega 1986, p. 110) but these nurses did not appear to be at any greater risk than other non-cancer nurses tested using the same instrument. The burnout scores of the cancer nurses in this study were also comparable to those of oncology nurse specialists reported by Yasko (1983). Factors that appeared to have a relationship with the score on the burnout scale included perceived support, level of role satisfaction, negative feelings about work as an oncology nurse, years in the role, and stress associated with the organization and physicians. Interestingly Ogle (1983) had previously described a study exploring burnout in oncology nurses in the hospital setting. Similarly, participants did perceive moderate burnout in their work experience and were aware of the stage of burnout they were experiencing within the framework of the Maslach Burnout Inventory (Maslach 1976).

In contrast, Bram & Kratz (1989) found that there were significant differences in the burnout scores between hospice-based nurses and hospital oncology nurses. They noted that both groups were subject to similar inherent job stresses. However, there were some differences in the demographics of each group. The hospice-based nurses tended to be older, married, more experienced and more academically trained. More hospice nurses perceived communication with administration to be good and felt that they had a greater sense of control over decision-making. It is difficult to draw any firm conclusions from a study based in the United States using 57 nurses. However, Bram & Kratz (1989) do suggest practical implications of providing support within the work environment, and this call is echoed in all research and discussion papers related to stress, burnout and cancer nursing.

Work-related stress was also explored in a research paper by Herschbach (1992). Physicians and nurses working with patients with cancer were compared with those working with patients in cardiac, intensive care or surgical units. A large sample (299 physicians and 592 nurses from 54 institutions) completed a specifically designed questionnaire about the emotional or physical distress caused by each of 64 situations. The researcher concluded that, although the degree of work-related stress was comparable across groups, the physicians and nurses from oncology settings experienced more feelings of emotional involvement and self-doubt.

The majority of research studies, including that of Ullrich & Fitzgerald (1990), which described the stress experienced by physicians and nurses in the cancer ward, have utilized structured tools or measures to determine levels of stress and burnout and factors (personality, intrinsic job related and work environment) that influence the experience of stress and burnout. The positivist approach has been the most prevalent model utilized in nursing research (Munhall 1982) and emphasis on it has represented a period of evolution. Having always been influenced by the 'philosophical underpinnings' of the time, nurses have tended to study within the paradigms of other disciplines and their theories have reflected a range of perspectives (Meleis 1985). The emphasis in nursing research on measurement, prediction and causal inference does not easily fit a nursing world with a broadly humanistic philosophy (Corner 1991, Munhall 1982). While these research studies have contributed to our understanding of stress and burnout within cancer care, they have continued to separate and compartmentalize stress from the everyday practice of cancer nurses and the central values of cancer nursing.

More recently qualitative research has offered an insight into a different facet of the cancer nursing experience (e.g. Pearce 1997). Broadly, a qualitative perspective oriented, as Benoliel (1984) explains, 'toward the unique nature of human thoughts, behaviours, negotiations and institutions under different sets of historical and environmental circumstances' (p. 7), has been used to focus on the meanings and experiences of what cancer nurses constitute as stressful. Pearce (1997) describes what her informants said constituted stress in cancer nursing. This incorporated the role of boundaries, 'difficult' relationships with patients and colleagues, the sense of not being 'good enough' as individual carers and as a service, the importance of time as a resource, not feeling valued or cared for, and the role of making sense and gaining some sense of mastery over the cancer nursing experience (Pearce 1997). These themes, developed through hermeneutic enquiry, have parallels with previous work in as much as the hospice nurses in Bram & Kratz's (1989) study experienced less dissonance than hospital-based oncology nurses between their perceived ideal job and the job they were actually doing.

Overall, the picture that emerges from the research and literature related to stress and burnout, and the emotional labour of cancer nursing is mixed. However, it is possible to extract some key issues that are worthy of debate within the specialty and necessitate further research. It can be contended that cancer nurses form special attachments with patients and their families, and experience feelings of emotional involvement. The stress associated with cancer nursing is intricately bound with the values, such as holism, that cancer nurses hold as central to the specialty. For example, not being able to provide 'good enough' care or a 'good enough' service (Pearce 1997) contributes to the dissonance that cancer nurses can potentially experience when the reality of their everyday practice is incongruent with the expectations of the individual nurse and those espoused by the specialty itself. The experience of stress also appears to centre on organizational job issues (e.g. staffing levels, interprofessional care, management support) and the nature of cancer care work (e.g. caring for patients with an uncertain future, maintaining the balance between hope and realism, contending with advancing technologies in our understanding of cancer, managing symptoms of cancer and its treatment, sometimes often intractable and chronic, etc.). Cancer nurses have acknowledged through conferences, papers and research, and in their day-to-day work environment, the importance of support and the need for cancer nursing to be valued. What research and cancer nurses themselves have yet to delineate with clarity is how this can be achieved, what support is effective and how can it be evaluated, and how, why, when and from whom do cancer nurses need to feel valued.

Maslach's (1976) original research noted the negative consequences of stress and burnout on the quality of services to patients and clients. Bram & Kratz (1989) describe how professionals (including lawyers, prison wardens, psychologists and psychiatric nurses) interviewed by Maslach distanced themselves to cope with the stress of their jobs. Strategies included being cynical and negative towards clients, physically distancing themselves in encounters with clients through lack of eye contact or minimal conversation, spending less time with patients and more socializing with colleagues, and 'going by the book' rather than responding to the uniqueness of the individual (Bram & Kratz 1989). Similarly nurses with higher burnout scores committed more serious job errors and tended to be more neglectful in their care (Jones 1980). Presently there is no evidence of the direct effects of burnout in cancer nursing for patient care, but many cancer nurses could offer examples of when they themselves had offered or witnessed unsatisfactory care that could be attributed to stress.

SUPPORT AND CANCER NURSING

The issue of support for cancer nurses and cancer nursing is embedded in the desire to facilitate the delivery of individualized and effective practice which, it has been argued, is the essence of cancer nursing. This issue is a wide-ranging one and can be addressed by examining and offering practical suggestions in relation to the organization and management of cancer care, education for cancer nursing, and research innovations within the specialty. Within the context of this chapter we will explore the issues of mentorship and clinical supervision.

Clinical supervision and mentorship

Morton-Cooper & Palmer (1993) argue that support is about 'being sensitive to the human dynamics that surround us. It is also about allowing individuals to be self-directive and assisting them to manage the change process for themselves' (p. 34). Clinical supervision and mentoring are suggested as strategies to support practising cancer nurses. The challenge when considering these is to distinguish the rhetoric from the pragmatics in order to offer a practical and coherent approach to a practice-based specialty.

It seems essential to identify what is meant by both mentorship and clinical supervision before considering their relevance to cancer nursing practice. Morton-Cooper & Palmer (1993) suggest that 'mentoring concerns the building of a dynamic relationship in which the personal characteristics, philosophies and priorities of the individual members interact to influence in turn the nature, direction and duration of the resulting, eventual partnership' (p. 59), and a mentoring relationship is one that 'is enabling and cultivating; a relationship that assists in empowering an individual within the working environment' (p. 59). Butterworth (1992) argues that mentors are seen as sharing experiences, offering the best way of approaching an issue, facilitating intellectual and personal growth, and helping with adaptation to new situations and challenges. The mentor has both an educative and supportive role; as Bond & Holland (1997) affirm, mentors are experienced practitioners who 'nurture and guide students in clinical placements' (p. 21).

There is an emerging literature related to both clinical supervision and mentoring. Butterworth (1992) posits a number of influences that have led nursing to look in the direction of supervision. These influences include the de-medicalization of nursing, the extension and expansion of nurses' role in all contexts of healthcare, and the emotional costs of nursing work (Butterworth 1992). More specifically Bond & Holland (1997) discuss factors that have contributed to the impetus towards clinical supervision in nursing in the UK. They contend that these developments

include 'broad organizational changes; policy directives; concerns about accountability; quality initiatives for improving standards of care; concepts of empowerment and partnership integrated into nursing philosophy; education drives
towards reflective practice; concern about practitioner health and preventing
burnout; and increased value on therapeutic interventions and the concomitant
need for self-awareness' (Bond & Holland 1997, p. 32). These are issues equally
relevant to nurses outside the UK. Hence, as Butterworth (1992) argues, models of
clinical supervision and mentorship can be developed in nursing which will 'protect and improve clinical practice and give nursing the necessary support it needs
to mature into greater independence' (p. 5).

Cancer nursing is also exposed to the same influences; the extensions and
expansions of the cancer nursing role, and the emotional labour and stress of
cancer nursing work, mean that the specialty also needs to discuss and evaluate
models of supportive practice that will facilitate the development and practice
of individual cancer nurses and the practice of the specialty.

The needs of practitioners in the transition phase after the completion of pre-
registration education or a change in area of clinical practice, for example a move
into the cancer nursing arena, have been a force in the development of mentorship
schemes. Cancer nurses need to consider how best to support those practitioners
who chose to enter the specialty of cancer nursing or who change their focus of
practice, for example from involvement in cancer screening to community-based
cancer nursing. It is beyond the scope of this text to review and evaluate
approaches to mentorship and the reader is referred to the texts of Butterworth &
Faugier (1992) and Morton-Cooper & Palmer (1993) for more indepth analysis and
examples of schemes in action. However, the potential value of mentorship to cancer nursing lies in creating a supportive environment for neophyte cancer nurses.
The best way to deal with burnout, Hawkins & Shohet (1989) suggest, is prevention. Perhaps more importantly, supporting the new cancer nurse in a systematic
rather than haphazard way means that it is possible to harness, release and
develop the skills required to enjoy cancer nursing as a rewarding area of practice.

Central to the difference between clinical supervision and mentorship in nursing
are the notions of mutual exchange and power. Butterworth (1992) suggests that
clinical supervision is based on mutual exchange, while Bond & Holland (1997)
note that there is less of a power divide in clinical supervision compared with
mentorship. Faugier (1992) continues the debate and stresses that clinical supervision should be about empowerment and not control. Notwithstanding this, the key
issue is that both approaches will provide the cancer nurse with opportunities for
support and development. As Bond & Holland (1997) eloquently explain, the differences are ones of emphasis in the educative and supportive functions of each.

Clinical supervision, Bond & Holland (1997, p. 12) go on to explain, is 'regular,
protected time for facilitated indepth reflection on clinical practice. It aims to
enable the supervisee to achieve, sustain and creatively develop a high quality of
practice through the means of focused support and development.' Hawkins &
Shohet (1989) explain that the British Association of Counselling (1987) have stated
that the primary purpose of supervision is to protect the best interests of the client.
The aims of clinical supervision include the expansion of a knowledge base, the
development of clinical expertise, self-esteem and autonomy (Platt-Koch 1986).
However, presently there is limited evidence within nursing delineating the role of
clinical supervision (or mentorship) in reducing stress, preventing burnout, or promoting personal and professional growth. The contention is that supervision is a
vehicle for promoting and developing quality practice (Bond & Holland 1997,
Butterworth & Faugier 1992). As Johns (1995) suggests, reflecting values and personal knowledge enables a philosophy of care to become a reality, develops expertise, and challenges and enables practitioners to become open and curious about

their practice. Therefore, we concur with Booth (1992), who posits that clinical supervision has a part to play in support and stress reduction.

Cancer nurses then, as they contemplate approaches to clinical supervision and support, need to consider the place of the person with cancer in the debate and ensure that evaluation is central to the process. At a practical level the benefits of a practitioner-centred support system, that is regular, structured, valued and part of the everyday life of cancer nursing, appear straightforward. The importance, and perhaps the success, of any approach to support in cancer nursing is that the initiative reflects the local and national context in which cancer practice is delivered and that practitioners themselves are pivotal in the design and structuring of mentorship and clinical supervision support systems. There are a variety of approaches to clinical supervision in nursing and other helping professions described by authors such as Hawkins & Shohet (1989), Butterworth & Faugier (1992) and Bond & Holland (1997). There are, however, few guidelines about setting up a clinical supervision system although general principles are offered by Kohner (1994), Swain (1995) and the United Kingdom Central Council (1996). Simply, Bond & Holland (1997) afford a six-stage framework – information sharing; skills training; decision about mode (e.g. one to one or group supervision); pilot, evaluate and redesign; and establish and monitor – that is helpful for those setting out on the process of clinical supervision.

The potential lies within the specialty to support the practice of cancer nursing not only through research and education but also by harnessing and utilizing the experience and energy of cancer nurses themselves. The value of clinical supervision is, we believe, in its commitment to sustaining, nurturing and developing nurses by fostering reflection on self and practice. Cancer nurses can learn from other disciplines and areas of nursing, and it would appear from the literature that debate, consensus and active involvement from practising cancer nurses are the first essential steps in the process of supervision. This process of support and supervision, it is argued, will underpin the evaluation, development and advancement of the specialty of cancer nursing practice.

VISION FOR THE FUTURE

It is important that cancer nurses keep abreast of developments and medical progress to enable them to provide professional cancer nursing intervention. New methods of treatment may require specific knowledge, for instance in gene therapy, where nurses need to extend their knowledge of cell biology, genetics and genetic engineering. It is therefore vital that nurses are given an opportunity for continued education, either through enrolment on external courses or at their own place of work. Cancer nursing must be able to believe in the possibilities of cancer care; reflection on different actions and situations is one form of care development and something that every nurse should consider practising. Patients will, in the future, increasingly be nursed in a non-institutional setting, partly due to the wider choice of options but perhaps also because of financial restraints. New forms of care and increased cooperation between primary and institutional care will therefore be necessary.

Russel (1991) states that we have to stop trying to define nursing or attempting to develop definitive role statements and instead 'move forward, with confidence, into the future' and, in addition, seek the answer to a number of questions: 'What do we want nursing to be?', 'How do we want to practice nursing in the future?', 'Where do we want to practice nursing?' and, 'How can we achieve changes in nursing and in nursing practice that we, the nursing profession, see as necessary?' (pp. 90–91). Russel believes that, in seeking the answers to these questions, we should strive to develop our own strategies for change so that the practice of nursing becomes what we, the members of that profession, want it to be. Is this way of thinking also going to lead to a new era of cancer nursing care? As European nurses we must also try to collaborate, despite cultural and language differences, so that developments in cancer nursing practice result in improved outcomes for persons with cancer and their families.

REFERENCES

American Nurses Association 1985 Proceedings from the Congress for Nursing Practice. The Clinical Nurse Specialist October 1985

Anderson J L 1989 The nurse's role in cancer rehabilitation. Review of the literature. Cancer Nursing 12(2):85–94

Artinian B M 1995 Risking involvement with cancer patients. Western Journal of Nursing Research 17(3):292–304

Athlin E, Furaker C, Jansson L, Noreberg A 1993 Application of primary nursing within a team setting in the hospice care of cancer patients. Cancer Nursing 16(5):388–397

Benner P, Wrubel J 1989 The primacy of caring. Addison-Wesley, Menlo Park, California

Benoliel J 1984 Advancing nursing science: qualitative approaches. Western Journal of Nursing Research 6(3):1–8

Bolund C 1990 Crisis and coping – learning to live with cancer. In: Veronesi U, Holland J C, Zittoun R (eds) European School of Oncology, Milan, p 13

Bourhis R Y, Roth S, MacQueen G 1989 Communication in the hospital setting: a survey of medical and everyday language use amongst patients, nurses and doctors. Social Science and Medicine 28(4):339–346

Blumberg B, Flaherty M, Lewis J (eds) 1980 Coping with cancer: a resource for the health professional. Bethesda, Maryland: National Cancer Institute

Bond M, Holland S 1997 Skills of clinical supervision for nurses. Open University Press, Buckingham

Booth K 1992 Providing support and reducing stress: a review of the literature. In: Butterworth T, Faugier J (eds) Clinical supervision and mentorship in nursing. Stanley Thornes, Cheltenham, UK, p 50

Bram P J, Kratz L F 1989 A study of burnout in nurses working in hospice and hospital oncology setting. Oncology Nursing Forum 16(4):555–560

Brandt B 1991 Information needs and selected variables in patients receiving brachytherapy. Oncology Nursing Forum 18:1221–1227

British Association of Counselling 1987 Cited in: Hawkins P, Shohet R 1989 Supervision in the helping professions. Open University Press, Milton Keynes, pp 41–54

Butterworth T 1992 Clinical supervision as an emerging idea in nursing. In: Butterworth T, Faugier J (eds) Clinical supervision and mentorship in nursing. Stanley Thornes, Cheltenham, UK, p 3

Butterworth T, Faugier J (eds) 1992 Clinical supervision and mentorship in nursing. Stanley Thornes, Cheltenham, UK

Cameron-Traub E 1991 An evolving discipline. In: Gray G, Pratt R (eds) Towards a discipline of nursing. Churchill Livingstone, Melbourne, p 31

Carson M, Williams T, Everett A, Barker S 1997 The nurse's role in the multidisciplinary team. European Journal of Palliative Care 4(3):96–98

Casselith B, Lusk E, Bodenheimer B 1985 Chemotherapy toxicity – the relationship between the patients' pretreatment expectations and post-treatment results. American Journal of Clinical Oncology 8:419–425

Cella D 1993 Quality of life as an outcome of cancer treatment. In: Groenwald S, Hansen Frogge M, Goodman M, Henke Yarbo C (eds) Cancer nursing: principles and practice, 3rd edn. Jones and Bartlett, Boston, p 197

Chinn P L, Jacobs M K 1987 Theory and nursing, 2nd edn. C V Mosby, St Louis

Clarke J B, Wheeler S J 1992 A view of the phenomenon of caring in nursing practice. Journal of Advanced Nursing 17:1283–1290

Cody W 1994 Nursing theory-guided practice: what it is and what it is not. Nursing Science Quarterly 7(4):144–145

Cody W, Mitchell G 1992 Parse's theory as a model for practice: the cutting edge. Advanced Nursing Science 15(2):52–65

Cohn K H 1982 Chemotherapy from an insider's perspective. Lancet i:1006–1009

Corner J 1991 In search of more complete answers to research questions. Quantitative versus qualitative research methods: is there a way forward. Journal of Advanced Nursing 16:718–727

Corner J 1997 Beyond survival rates and side effects: cancer nursing as therapy. Cancer Nursing 20(1):3–11

Delvaux N, Razaavi D, Farvacques C et al 1988 Cancer care – a stress for health professionals. Social Science and Medicine 27(2):159–166

Derdiarian A 1987a Informational needs of recently diagnosed cancer patients: a theoretical framework. Cancer Nursing 10(2):107–115

Derdiarian A 1987b Informational needs of recently diagnosed cancer patients: method and description. Cancer Nursing 10(3):156–163

Dodd M 1982 Assessing patient self-care for side effects of cancer chemotherapy – part 1. Cancer Nursing 5(6):447–451

Dorsett D 1993 Quality of care. In: Groenwald S, Hansen Frogge M, Goodman M, Henke Yarbo C (eds) Cancer nursing: principles and practice, 3rd edn. Jones and Bartlett, Boston, p 1453

Ersser S 1991 A search for the therapeutic dimensions of nurse–patient interaction. In: McMahon R, Pearson A (eds) Nursing as Therapy. Chapman and Hall, London, p 43

Faugier J 1992 The supervisory relationship. In: Butterworth T, Faugier J (eds) Clinical supervision and mentorship in nursing. Stanley Thornes, Cheltenham, UK, p 18

Faulkner A, Maguire P 1994 Talking to cancer patients and their relatives. Oxford Medical Publications, Oxford

Felstein M A, Gemma P B 1995 Oncology nurses and chronic grief. Cancer Nursing 18(3):228–236

Felton B J, Revenson T A 1984 Coping with chronic illness: a study of illness controllability and the influence of coping strategies on psychological adjustment. Journal of Consulting Clinical Psychology 52:343–353

Fernsler J 1986 A comparison of patient and nurse perceptions of patients' self-care deficits associated with cancer chemotherapy. Cancer Nursing 9(2):50–57

Ferrell B, O`Neil-Page E 1993 Continuity of care. In: Groenwald S, Hansen Frogge M, Goodman M, Henke Yarbo C (eds) Cancer nursing: principles and practice, 3rd edn. Jones and Bartlett, Boston, p 1346

Forrest D 1989 The experience of caring. Journal of Advanced Nursing 14:815–823

Gaut D A 1993 Caring: a vision of wholeness for nursing. Journal of Holistic Nursing 11(2):164–171

Glaus A 1993 Quality of life – a measure of the quality of nursing care? Supportive Care in Cancer 1(3):119–123

Goodman, M 1989 Managing the side effects of chemotherapy. Seminars in Oncology Nursing 5(2) (suppl 1):29–52

Grahn G, Johnson J 1990 Learning to cope and living with cancer: learning needs assessment in cancer education. Scandinavian Journal of Caring Sciences 4:173–175

Graydon J, Galloway S, Palmer-Wickham S et al 1997 Information needs of women during early treatment for breast cancer. Journal of Advanced Nursing 26:59–64

Griffin A 1993 Holism in nursing: its meaning and value. British Journal of Nursing 2(6):310–312

Halldórsdóttir S, Hamrin E 1997 Caring and uncaring encounters within nursing and health care from the cancer patient's perspective. Cancer Nursing 20(2):120–128

Hawkins P, Shohet R 1989 Supervision in the helping professions. Open University Press, Milton Keynes

Herschbach P 1992 Work-related stress specific to physicians and nurses working with cancer patients. Journal of Psychosocial Oncology 10(2):79–99

Hogan C 1997 Cancer nursing: the art of symptom management. Oncology Nursing Forum 24(8):1335–1341

Hooker L 1997 Information needs of teenagers with cancer: developing a tool to explore the perceptions of patients and professionals. Journal of Cancer Nursing 1(4):160–168

Jenkins J F, Ostchega Y 1986 Evaluation of burnout in oncology nurses. Cancer Nursing 9(3):108–116

Johns C 1995 The value of reflective practice of nursing. Journal of Clinical Nursing 4:23–30

Jones J 1980 Preliminary test manual for the staff burnout scale for health care professionals. London House Management Consultants, Illinois

Jourard S M 1971 The transparent self, 2nd edn. Van Nostrand Reinhold, New York

Kelly P 1992 Informational needs of individuals and families with hereditary cancers. Seminars in Oncology Nursing 8(7):288–292

Kohner N 1994 Clinical supervision in practice. Kings Fund Centre, London

Larson D G 1992 The challenge of caring in oncology nursing. Oncology Nursing Forum 19(6):857–861

Lazarus R S 1966 Psychological stress and the coping process. MacGraw-Hill, New York

Lazarus R S, Folkman S 1984 Stress, appraisal and coping. Springer, New York

Leininger M 1981 Caring: an essential human need: proceedings of the three national conferences. M Slack, Thorofare, New Jersey

Leininger M 1988 Leininger's theory of nursing: cultural care diversity and universality. Nursing Science Quarterly 1:152–160

Luker K A, Beaver K, Leinster S J, Glynn Owens R, Degner L F, Sloan J 1995 The information needs of women newly diagnosed with breast cancer. Journal of Advanced Nursing 22:134–141

Luker K A, Beaver K, Leinster S J, Glynn Owens R 1996 Information needs and sources of information for women with breast cancer: a follow up study. Journal of Advanced Nursing 23:487–495

Lützén K, Barbosa da Silva A 1995 Delineating the scientific domain of nursing in Sweden – some relevant issues. Vardi i Norden 15(1):4–7

Mahon S 1991 Managing the psychosocial consequences of cancer recurrence: implications for nurses. Oncology Nursing Forum 18(3):577–583

McElroy A M 1982 Burnout – a review of the literature with application to cancer nursing. Cancer Nursing 5(3):211–217

Macguire J 1989 An approach to evaluating the introduction of primary nursing in an acute medical unit for the elderly. I – Principles and Practice. International Journal of Nursing Studies 26:243–251

Macleod Clark J 1982 Nurse/patient verbal interaction. PhD thesis, University of London, London

McMahon R, Pearson A (eds) 1991 Nursing as therapy. Chapman and Hall, London

Maslach C 1976 Burned out. Human Behavior 5(9):16–22

Maslach C, Pines A 1977 The burn-out syndrome in the day care setting. Child Care Quarterly 6:110–113

Meleis A 1985 Theoretical nursing: development and progress. Lippincott, Philadelphia

Mishel M, Hotsetter T, King B, Graham V 1984 Predictors of psychosocial adjustment in patients newly diagnosed with gynaecological cancer. Cancer Nursing 7:291–299

Mitchell G W, Glicksman A S 1977 Cancer patients: knowledge and attitudes. Cancer 40(1):61–66

Morse W, Werner J 1988 Individualization of patient care using Orem's theory. Cancer Nursing 11(3):195–202

Morton-Cooper A, Palmer A 1993 Mentoring and preceptorship: a guide to support roles in clinical practice. Blackwell Science, Oxford

Muetzel P 1988 Therapeutic nursing. In: Pearson A (ed) Primary nursing: nursing in the Burford and Oxford nursing development units. Croom Helm, London, p 89

Muldary T 1983 Burnout and health professionals: manifestations and management. Appleton-Century-Crofts, Nowalk, Connecticut

Munhall P 1982 Nursing philosophy and nursing research: in apposition or opposition? Nursing Research 31(3):176–177

Newlin N J, Wellisch D K 1978 The oncology nurse: life on an emotional roller coaster. Cancer Nursing 1(6):447–449

Northouse P G, Northouse L L 1987 Communication and cancer: issues confronting patients, health care professionals, and family members. Journal of Psychosocial Oncology 5(3):17–46

Oberst M T 1978 Priorities in cancer nursing research. Cancer Nursing 1(4):281–290

Ogle M E 1983 Stages of burnout among oncology nurses in hospital settings. Oncology Nursing Forum 10(1):31–34

O'Malley J, Loveridge C, Cummings S 1989 The new nursing organization. Nursing Management 20:29–33

Orem D 1985 Nursing: concepts of practice, 3rd edn. McGraw-Hill, New York

Padilla G, Grant M 1985 Quality of life as a cancer nursing outcome variable. Advances in Nursing Science 8(1):45–60

Pearce S 1997 The experience of stress for cancer nurses: a heideggerian phenomenological approach. MSc thesis, University of London, London

Pelusi J 1997 The lived experience of surviving breast cancer. Oncology Nursing Forum 24(8):1343–1353

Peters-Golden H 1982 Breast cancer: varied perceptions of social support in the illness experience. Social Science and Medicine 16(4):483–491

Platt-Koch L M 1986 Clinical supervision for psychiatric nurses. Journal of Psychological Nursing 26(1):7–15

Powell J 1991 Reflection and the evaluation of practice: prerequisites for therapeutic practice. In: McMahon R, Pearson A (eds) Nursing as therapy. Chapman and Hall, London, p 26

Pyles S H, Stern P 1983 Discovery of nursing gestalt in critical care nursing: the importance of the grau gorilla syndrome. Image: Journal of Nursing Scholarship 15(2):51–57

Reville B, Almadrones L 1989 Continuous infusion chemotherapy in the ambulatory setting: the nurse's role in patient selection and education. Oncology Nursing Forum 16(4):529–535

Rieker P, Clarke E, Fogelberg P 1992 Perceptions of quality of life and quality of care for patients with cancer receiving biological therapy. Oncology Nursing Forum 19(3):433–440

Rittman M, Paige P, Rivera J, Sutphin L, Godown I 1997 Phenomenological study of nurses caring for dying patients. Cancer Nursing 20(2):115–119

Roach M S 1987 The human art of caring. Canadian Hospital Association, Ottawa

Robinson L 1994 The experience of cancer recurrence: a phenomenological study. MSc thesis, University of London, London

Russel L 1991 Are we asking the right questions? In: Gray G, Pratt R (eds) Towards a discipline of nursing. Churchill Livingstone, Melbourne, p 73

Selye H 1956 The stress of life. MacGraw-Hill, New York

Siehl S 1982 The clinical nurse specialist in oncology. Nursing Clinics of North America 17(4):753–761

Silver R L, Wortman W B 1980 Coping with undesirable life events. In: Garber J, Seligman M E P (eds) Human helplessness: theory and applications. Academic Press, New York

Smith G S, Richardson A 1996 Development of nursing documentation for use in the outpatient oncology setting. European Journal of Cancer Care 5(4):225–232

Smith M 1994 Beyond the threshold: nursing practice in the next millennium. Nursing Science Quarterly 7(1):6–7

Spiegel D, Bloom J R, Yalom I 1981 Group support for patients with metastatic cancer: a randomized outcome study. Archives of General Psychiatry 38(5):527–533

Spielberger C D, Gorsch R L, Lushene R E 1983 Manual for the state–trait anxiety inventory. Counselling Psychological Press, Palo Alto, California

Stotland E, Mathews K E, Sherman S E et al 1978 Empathy, fantasy and helping. Sage Publications, Beverly Hills, California

Stowers S 1983 Nurses cry too, being exposed to grief and loss – how we deal with our own grief. Nursing Management 14:63–64

Stromberg M 1986 Health promotion behaviours in ambulatory cancer patients: fact or fiction? Oncology Nursing Forum 13:37–43

Swain G 1995 Clinical supervision: the principles and process. Community Practitioners and Health Visitors Association, London

Tiffany R 1987 The development of cancer nursing as a speciality. International Nursing Review 34(2):35–39

Ullrich A, Fitzgerald P 1990 Stress experienced by physicians and nurses in the cancer ward. Social Science and Medicine 31(9):1013–1022

United Kingdom Central Council 1996 Position statement on clinical supervision for nursing and midwifery. UKCC for Nursing, Midwifery and Health Visiting, London

van Sevellen G, Leake B 1993 Burn-out in hospital nurses: a comparison of acquired immunodeficiency syndrome, oncology, general medical, and intensive care unit nurse samples. Journal of Professional Nursing 9(3):169–177

Watson J 1979 Nursing: the philosophy and science of caring. Little, Brown, Boston

Watson J 1985 Nursing: the philosophy and science of caring. Associated University Press, Colorado

Welch-McCaffrey D 1983 When it comes to cancer – think family. Nursing 13(12):32–35

Welch-McCaffrey D 1986 Role performance issues for oncology clinical nurse specialists. Cancer Nursing 9(6):287–294

Wengstrom Y, Haggmark C 1998 Assessing nursing problems of importance for the development of nursing care in a radiation therapy department. Cancer Nursing 21(1):50–56

Wilkinson S 1991 Factors which influence how nurses communicate with cancer patients. Journal of Advanced Nursing 16:677–688

Yano B 1977 Special needs of oncology nursing. Journal of Practical Nursing 6(3):28–30

Yasko J 1983 Variables which predict burnout experienced by oncology nurse specialists. Cancer Nursing 6:109–116

Yasko J, Rust D 1989 Trends in chemotherapy administration. Seminars in Oncology Nursing 5(2) (suppl 1):3–7

Leadership and management: influencing the shape of advanced cancer nursing practice

Agnes Glaus   Phyllis Campbell   Nora Kearney
Alison Richardson

INTRODUCTION

This chapter deals with aspects of nursing management and leadership. It will cover, in varying degrees of detail, organizational and economic issues, the emotional costs of nursing, recruitment and retention, continuing professional development, the role of management in implementing research in practice and quality assurance. These issues are covered here, as they cannot be seen separately from advanced cancer nursing practice. They present the foundation for its developments and achievements.

It has been claimed that the emphasis on reducing healthcare costs in current health care threatens the delivery of quality cancer care (Mooney 1997). In addition to this statement the US Oncology Nursing Society also contends that nurses who have undertaken specific education in cancer care are essential to the provision of quality cancer care throughout all phases of the cancer experience. In most European countries this standard has yet to be achieved and it is only through quality management of cancer nursing services that it will be reached. The developing role of nurse managers in oncology is a difficult and multifaceted one, and requires a range of skills and knowledge to ensure the value of nursing is reflected in contemporary cancer care.

Current restructuring of care is accelerating the shift in cancer care from hospital and clinic to home, yet the provision of services by oncology nurses in such a setting is severely limited. Frameworks for cancer nursing care delivery that are capable of recognizing evolving care contexts need to be established and then maintained. A framework can be used to underpin the planning, delivery and evaluation of care. This should be capable of reflecting the totality of care and treatment provided at each stage of a particular cancer pathway, thus making it necessary to move beyond traditional institutional boundaries.

Nurse managers should build on developments that have already taken place, by continually reviewing teams and skill-mix to support role developments wherever they can benefit patients. Opportunities for role development (whether it concerns extension or expansion) need to be carefully assessed, and risks and benefits properly considered. The future of such cancer nursing practice roles depends not only on the demonstration of positive quality and cost outcomes for patients with cancer, but on definitions of the specific components of nursing practice that lead to positive outcomes in cancer care. To further understanding of the meaning of cancer nursing practice and its potential contribution to shaping the future of cancer care, the contributions of all nursing practice roles, whether established or evolving, must be evaluated. Verification of cancer nursing's contribution to improved quality of life requires assessment of the structures, processes and outcomes related to cancer nursing practice. The knowledge gained from such inquiry can be used to improve the organization, delivery and resourcing of cancer care services and to enhance the practice, education and research activities of nurses.

ECONOMIC AND EMOTIONAL COST OF NURSING

The cost and value of nursing

Everything has a price, and the same applies to nursing. Money is, and will remain, a major challenge for the nursing profession. The growing preoccupation with economic constraints, over quality issues of caring, gives cause for concern. One of the greatest problems in nursing is the fact that it has, so far, failed to show its financial value. This is best reflected in the fact that the most sophisticated healthcare systems do not explicitly acknowledge that the cost of nursing care is built in to overall care costs. Whilst nursing care is implicitly incorporated into any cost equation, the explicit financial value remains unassessed. Usually, nursing costs are covered in relation to the cost per day of being in a hospital bed, and they remain embedded in an overall budget. True economic worth is not measured and there is no basis for pricing. Nursing seems not to be seen as holding revenue-producing potential but is treated rather as 'generating expenses only' (Hendricks 1997). Yet, more than half of all National Health Service (NHS) staff in England are nurses, and nursing services (Dean 1992) absorb a quarter of all health service expenditure. In Australia, 60–70% of the hospital staff budget will go towards the cost of nursing care (Australian Institute of Health and Welfare 1994). These facts reflect the importance of nursing and the need to determine the cost of its services accurately. In the past, it was expected that nursing care would be provided in the spirit of a dedicated service rather than for financial gain. It was assumed that caring was incongruent with the objectivity required for monetary compensation (Hendricks 1997). Today, caregivers and consumers are confronted with the question of whether they are ready to value nursing care in real economic terms and the community has to decide whether it both wants and can afford such services.

Even though many oncology nurses still want to practise in the spirit of a dedicated service, today it is clear that the workload of nurses needs to be assessed in order to assure and justify adequate staffing levels. The method of funding a nursing service will influence an institution's ability to administer 'quality care'. Costs have significance because the realization of goals and the attainment and maintenance of standards are in direct proportion to the adequacy of available resources (Pfefferkorn & Rovetta 1940). This observation from the first half of the twentieth century remains relevant, and thus a major challenge for the present. If nursing is to be offered as a separate, identifiable identity to the consumer, nursing costs need to be defined and justified. This is possible only if nurse managers can act independently to obtain and analyse relevant data in order to estimate costs and benefits. New systems for the measurement of the type and load of nursing activities will help to make nursing economically visible – even though this might also add new problems, because in the future there will be less, rather than more, money, available for healthcare services.

Measuring workload and calculating the cost of nursing

Nurses in administrative positions have been concerned by system cost and use of resources for a long time. An impressive diversity appears to exist concerning nursing resources between European countries. An international study by Reid & Melaugh (1987) assessed the number of professional nurses (with professional qualifications) per 10 000 population in different countries. England (26.9) and France (28.7) fared very much worse than did Sweden (67.2) or Switzerland (63.1). Northern Ireland (47.7) and Scotland (57.8) had over twice as many nurses per 10 000 population as had England and Wales (23.51) at that time. From this study, however, the question of whether the quality of care is better in the countries with higher staff levels, or whether staff resources are being less efficiently used, cannot be answered, even though it might be assumed that such profound differences may have a strong impact. In all countries, a dearth of financial resources, increases in complex nursing activities, daily variation in workload, and shorter hospital stays which generate a higher level of acuity, were among the factors that promoted the call for more objective instruments, in order to collect nursing cost data and allocate nursing personnel (Thibault et al 1990).

An investigation carried out in Holland showed that nursing workload in oncology is not a static feature and that its documentation may reflect developments and changes over time, which are crucial to nursing. A 14-year study revealed a significant increase in workload, along with changes in medical treatment (Van Dam 1990). In this longitudinal study, a classification system, comprising seven categories, was used daily by nurses to assess the current situation. Expenditure of time varied from 30 min for category 1 (the patient is ambulatory and self-supporting) to 240 min for category 7 (the patient is undergoing intensive treatment and requires total nursing care). In relation to the direct care, a number of constant workload factors was added. Even though the method of measurement used can be criticized, and might even be considered outdated today, the study was able to show that the staffing system needed to be flexible in order to respond both to daily changing demands and also to changes in medical treatment strategies over time. The implications for cost-effectiveness fail to result in adaptations to nursing. The researcher assumed that, in 1990, the increased workload in oncology in Holland had kept only partially abreast of the increase in staff required to manage the workload.

Workload measurement instruments, such as GRASP (Meyers 1985) or PNR (Prediction of Nursing Requirements) (Kuhn 1980), usually measure the time required to care for a patient based on a validated standard time of care, which permits a quantification of the number of people required to carry out the predictable activities over a determined period of time. Systems are used either on a daily basis, to adjust the basic team according to the variations in patients' needs, or they help nurse administrators to use such data retrospectively to analyse trends on an annual basis and correlate with indicators such as overtime, absenteeism or use of resource personnel (Thibault et al 1990). Such systems also facilitate the achievement of balanced workload between teams and budget planning. Data collection allows analysis of developments or changes in nursing care over time and might induce adjustments concerning skill-mix or educational needs.

It is generally acknowledged that in nursing care many activities are not visible, which presents a problem in terms of measurement. For example, nurses co-ordinate multi-professional activities, teach students, do administrative work or help with certain non-nursing tasks. As invisible work is not non-existent work, a workload measurement instrument must pay regard to such a reality. Provision must be made for both tangible and intangible determinants associated with nursing. Instruments can have limitations as regards validity and reliability but also in relation to the context in which they can be used with confidence. An instrument therefore should not be seen as independent from either the philosophy of care or management style of the institution.

Several patient classification systems have been developed in the past years for specific populations, such as psychiatric, medical-surgical, adult care, intensive care, neonatal care or new born nursery units (Lovett, Wagner & McMillan 1991). Acuity systems in oncology were expected to assist with: measurement of patient care needs, recommendation of daily staff allocations, staff scheduling for a defined period of time, budgetary and fiscal management and costing out of nursing services (Lovett, Wagner & McMillan 1991). One patient classification system that has been designed specifically for oncology patients is the Oncology Patient Classification System (OPCS) described by Magnusson (1985). In this system, acuity levels are determined by assessing the amount of nursing time involved in direct and indirect care for the patients and their families, and are based on indicators related to medical diagnoses. The OPCS may provide a better indication of actual requirements for patient care in oncology than other systems, such as patient classification by diagnosis-related groups. Variations in patient acuity and greater use of hospital resources, specifically observed with variations during cancer treatment, are not fully accounted for in the diagnosis-related groups' payment rate (Yasko & Fleck 1984). The OPCS categorizes patients by acuity of illness into five levels of care required within 24 hours. The instrument, tested for validity and reliability, consists of 41 therapeutic indicators which are descriptive phrases representing clinical situations requiring nursing intervention. It is based on the case-mix model and is related to actual care requirement. The model permits the prediction of care for future patients and supports adequate staffing and budget planning. It has been recommended for its ability to reflect nursing and hospital costs (Magnusson 1985).

The OPCS was used as a base for the development of the Paediatric Haematology Oncology Acuity Tool, which, in contrast, is based on nursing diagnoses, reflecting the cognitive basis of nursing practice and patient care (Lovett, Wagner & McMillan 1991). The Medical Oncology Patient Acuity Tool and the Surgical Oncology Patient Acuity Tool are also based on nursing diagnoses, and actually interface with nursing standards of care (Busch et al 1994). Two further systems have been developed for patients with bone marrow transplantation (Busch & McMillan 1993) and for those being nursed on a critical care unit (oncology) (Marsee, Busch & McMillan 1995). These systems have shown to be reliable and valid for use in these specific circumstances.

The case-mix finding model is another way of determining the costs of nursing. It attempts to separate out medical and nursing care needs and environmental factors, and establishes the visibility and economical value of nursing care (Hendricks 1997). Here, nursing is viewed as a product, which requires a clear basis for its pricing. Case-mix information is combined with client dependency or nursing intensity measures, which allow the nurse manager to determine average costs according to the related classification system. It has been suggested, however, that the accuracy of the relationship between acuity levels and staffing might be questioned (Stefan, Gillies & Biordi 1992). A patient's acuity level might be low physically, but high as a result of a deep emotional crisis, requiring intensive emotional support. A problem that might arise is the question of who defines the need for intensive emotional support and of whether the client or even the nurse is willing to accept that this support is not free of charge.

A model of assessing and measuring nursing care in German-speaking countries has been developed recently in Switzerland. The system is called LEP (Leistungserfassung in der Pflege), which roughly translates as 'documenting individual nursing services'. The system captures actual care requirements, measures the time involved and thus can calculate individual patient workload over a 24-hour period. The nursing activities are recorded daily after each shift for each patient by the attending nurses (a coded, computerized system). The total amount of work is then related to the number of staff available on the ward (individual, computerized registration), which reflects the ward situation and supports decisions concerning daily staff allocation. As the data available reflect the amount of care hours per individual patient, it might be used in future in relation to costing nursing services for individual patients. Data regarding workload and type of work over monthly, quarterly or annual periods also support budgetary and fiscal management.

The system is not based on a classification model, but is built on·categories of nursing activities, to which around 100 nursing tasks or activities are allocated. A standardized time factor is allocated to each activity. Table 3.1 presents the definitions, which relate to the 12 nursing categories (Mäder & Bamert 1994). An additional time factor is included in order to pay regard to indirect, invisible patient care, for example for the support of nursing students, handovers and coordinating activities. A retrospectively calculated coefficient between nursing activities and nursing staff hours available over the past 24 hours is used to express the workload situation on a ward (Mäder & Bamert 1994).

Historically, nurses have had difficulty in justifying the need for a higher staffing level in oncology in comparison with other areas of care. The LEP system, which also measures dimensions of psychological support, can now demonstrate anticipated staffing levels. For example, specific variables are available to document the workload induced by a psychological crisis, for example after breaking bad news. Specific variables like 'accompanying the dying' are available for inclusion to mirror the work situation realistically. These variables, however, are not specifically tailored to oncology nursing care but are also available for documenting the work of other (non-cancer care) patients. In some departments, the staffing level was assumed by nurses to be higher than could be demonstrated using LEP; in others it demonstrated a continuously lower level of workload. Figure 3.1 shows the percentage of nursing activities undertaken in a 23-bedded medical oncology ward according to the different nursing categories in a 900-bed teaching hospital in St Gallen, Switzerland (over a 1-year period). It also shows that, in addition to this information, the average number of nursing hours per patient over a defined period, the activities performed for each patient, the number of patient days, and the occupancy rate amongst other variables of interest

Table 3.1 Categories of nursing activities and number of variables allocated, as represented in the LEP system

Category	No. of nursing variables
1 Admissions, discharges	9
2 Movement	6
3 Physical hygiene	5
4 Eating and drinking	4
5 Elimination	7
6 Support/instruction/counselling	8
7 Nursing documentation	2
8 Discussions with other disciplines	4
9 Surveillance (monitoring)	2
10 Laboratory tests	3
11 Medications	7
12 Therapeutic interventions	15
13 Ward-specific variables	7

From Mäder & Bamert 1994, with permission.

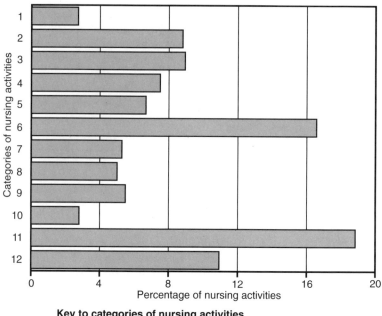

Key to categories of nursing activities

1	Admissions and discharges
2	Movement
3	Physical hygiene
4	Eating and drinking
5	Elimination
6	Support/instruction/counselling
7	Nursing documentation
8	Discussions with other disciplines
9	Surveillance (monitoring)
10	Laboratory tests
11	Medications
12	Therapeutic interventions

Additional information
Mean age of patients: 60.6 years
Average nursing care needed per patient day: 3.8 hours
Occupancy rate: 84.1%

Figure 3.1   Results of LEP statistical analysis for 1997 within a 23-bedded medical oncology ward (Kantonsspital St Gallen, Switzerland).

can be derived and analysed. In the hospital chosen for this illustration, staffing level does not now relate solely to a static number of nursing positions but rather represents a continuous process through which to allocate adequate human resources to the different patient areas, according to patient need. With the LEP system, individual patient care requirements over a 24-hour period are documented. The nursing management of a hospital of any size can obtain daily, weekly or monthly results from all departments in order to allocate human resources for understaffed or overstaffed units.

Even though the LEP system is still being refined, a continuing process is being led by a group of nursing and economic experts, and its future use seems promising. Meanwhile, the commercially available system is in use in approximately 50 Swiss hospitals and has been developed for different specialty areas, such as adult general nursing, intensive care, paediatric nursing, rehabilitation and psychiatry (Mayrhofer 1997). In other specialized areas, for example oncology, specific activities can be added to the system as unit-adjusted variables (activities). A further version of LEP is now being developed for patients with ambulatory care needs in outpatient departments or day-care units, as it is anticipated that in future a majority of patients will be treated on an outpatient basis. LEP has the potential to be developed for further fields.

A strength of the LEP system lies in the fact that nurses in the practice field, which helps ensure validity, have generated the data set. Ward sisters further check the validity and reliability of the data on a daily or weekly basis. Steps need to be undertaken continuously to test and support aspects of validity and reliability, such as training of new staff members, providing user conferences and providing regular discussions with nursing experts. This is crucial because all nurses need to document their activities thoroughly and according to the system-specific rules. Further work is needed in using data obtained to predict staffing that is sensitive to skill-mix. It has been demonstrated that a nurse with more training has a tendency to identify greater psychosocial need and can handle a larger workload (Halloran 1983). The LEP system does not yet differentiate between nurses with different levels of education, apart from the differentiation between registered nurses, students and new employees, whose working capacity is calculated at a reduced, standardized percentage.

Ethical and professional considerations with workload measurement

Independent of the type of workload measurement system, the interface between ethical and economic aspects requires discussion. The detailed assessment of nursing activities could result in a cost explosion. In this scenario, who decides about the type and amount of nursing care to be delivered? Will patients themselves or their insurance companies decide whether the nursing activities, including being supported emotionally, are worth the price? This not only presents a professional challenge but also might prove a burden on nurses who prefer to give human services without charging the patient. This requires refinements to the content of nursing education programmes, resulting in a deeper understanding of economic features. Further, some aspects, such as being involved emotionally in the patient's and the family's suffering, will never be visible within a record but will remain an essence of nursing.

Some criticism has been levelled at measurement systems generally. It has been expressed that too much paperwork has been created, with the implication that this has in relation to time, rather than devoting such time to delivering suitable care and that objective measurement is overvalued (Scher 1988). However, even though nurses' workload is a complex reality, which can be measured only imperfectly, valid administrative decisions can be supported with the help of these instruments.

EMOTIONAL COSTS OF NURSING CARE AND FINANCIAL CONSEQUENCES

Caring for patients with cancer involves many complicated human processes. It is difficult to articulate what happens between nurses and patients when they meet. Nurses deal with vulnerable individuals who experience dependency, fear and suffering, and might be confronted with potential death and dying. It is inevitable that in some circumstances the nurse becomes a companion. Campbell (1984) has characterized the nurse's role as one of the skilled companion and, in doing so, brings together the science and moral base of nursing practice. The ability to identify the needs of patients requires emotions. Empathy has been proposed to be the motivational base of helping (Hoffmann 1981). It comprises the recognition of what others are experiencing. Nurses experience empathetic distress if they recognize pain, fear and suffering in a patient. Only when they recognize that these feelings occur in the other person does sympathetic distress translate into helping action (Hoffmann 1981). The daily challenge for nurses, especially in oncology, is to recognize the feelings and pain in the other person but at the same time to remain aware of being a 'separate person'. Repeated identification with the severely ill patient may represent a danger in terms of 'overinvolvement', where the boundaries between self and others become blurred and where the helper may go to excessive lengths to control and dominate the situation to ensure that their own interests are protected (Benner & Wrubel 1989). Whether overinvolvement is the key to burnout syndrome, could not, however, be supported empirically.

Burnout syndrome has been defined by Maslach (1982) as 'the loss of human caring', accompanied by physical symptoms which may include stomach disorders, headaches, depression, fatigue, irritability, insomnia, rashes and exacerbation of chronic disease. Later, Benner & Wrubel (1989) defined burnout as 'the separation of caregiving and care and these authors associate it with the lack of meaningful distinctions' (p. 372). They describe it as a modern mistake to think that caring is the cause of burnout and that the cure is to protect oneself from caring. They see the loss of caring as 'sickness', accompanied by physical symptoms, and the return of caring as 'recovery'. In this sense, the meaning and the consequences of burnout in nurses are vital because they affect the essence of nursing, namely caring.

Meanwhile, it is well known that exhaustion of caregivers is dependent on many aspects other than just direct professional interactions with severely ill and dying patients and their relatives, for example institutional working conditions and the personal background of the caregiver (Alexander 1993, Astudillo & Mendinueta 1996). The multifactorial aetiology of the syndrome, which is only partially specific to the field of oncology, must challenge nurse managers to take preventive action. The concept of burnout is discussed in more detail in Chapter 2.

There is little scientific evidence to underpin the development of effective management strategies to prevent burnout. Nurse managers need to be alert to signs and symptoms, and to speak early with colleagues if there is concern. In oncology, it could be argued that it is more evident than elsewhere that nurse managers also need to be leaders, who give attention not only to 'how things get done' but also to 'what they mean to the person' who provides the service (Zaleznik 1977). Assessing workload and providing appropriate human resources as needed might represent a major supporting factor in the prevention of burnout syndrome. Lees (1990) identified lack of human resources as the most important stressor in 53 nurses on different wards. Recruitment, continuing education and staff retention play an important role and are described later in this chapter. Even though there is little scientific evidence, regular team support groups, which are supervised by an expert in psycho-oncology, are commonly practised in European countries and might be seen as preventive strategies. Reflecting on nurse–patient relationships and speaking about the experiences of cancer nursing in a protected environment can alleviate caregivers' suffering because it offers a possibility of releasing feelings, the opportunity of realizing overinvolvement, and the chance to experience strength through team spirit. As conflicts with physicians have also been identified as a major stressor in hospitals, the integration of physicians in such support groups might be recommended (Lees 1990, Ullrich 1990).

Today there is a continuing debate surrounding the question of who should pay for such support. The authors conclude from their experience, that it is very much in the interests of the hospital to support professional high-quality nursing in the emotionally challenging field of cancer care by providing psychological support for the nurses and physicians concerned. The time involved, however, might be financed by both parties, by the hospital and the nurse together. This not only makes the support sessions more precious, but can also be seen as developmental activity in relation to both one's professional and personal life.

LEADERSHIP

Already it is apparent that there are numerous factors that impinge on the management of cancer services, and it seems clear that to effect change requires leadership. Leadership must be seen as an integral component of the manager's role, particularly in the current climate of change within healthcare, irrespective of the domain of care. Given that nurses represent the largest group of healthcare professionals in cancer care, it is clear that the potential for effective leadership is enormous should nurses wish to accept this challenge. It has been argued that leadership is the first component of being an effective manager (Tappen 1989), yet access to leadership training is variable across Europe, although the King's Fund initiative in the UK is an excellent example of this. This has been extended to include a European Summer School for strategic leaders with a clinical background.

Leadership has been defined as the process of influencing others (Tannenbaum et al 1974) and as the ability to translate intention into reality and sustain it (Bennis & Nanus 1985). Through leadership, then, we attempt to influence others to ensure the optimal delivery of care in any situation whilst ensuring that nursing is recognized at a policy level. The development of these complex skills is unlikely to be inherent, and a number of theories and concepts have been postulated to explain how people can influence another's behaviour in a work situation (see Tappen 1989). However, on reviewing this literature, it is clear that no single theory can fully account for the complex and dynamic leadership skills that are required in managing an efficient cancer service. Despite this, however, the profile of a nurse leader could be said to have the following characteristics (King's Fund Management College 1995, p. 5):

- *A strategist – able to develop and implement strategy*

- *An environmentalist – able to adapt the organisation to a changing environment, looking at ways to make the organisation effective locally, and at ways of managing information*

- *A politically aware operator – able to work with national and local priorities and to use political awareness to the benefit of the organisation*

- *A confident leader – able to contribute fully to board level working, and to the professional development of nursing; able to lead beyond hierarchy in complex organisations. Has well-developed process consultancy skills.*

- *A sense of purpose – self aware and able to recognise and maximise personal impact, comfortable with self and able to express themselves through their work.*

If we are to continue the development of cancer nursing, it is vital that we should begin to identify leaders in the field of cancer nursing across Europe. It is surprising that in the specialty of cancer nursing, which is claimed to be one of the most developed specialties in Europe, there remains a lack of leadership at both the national and European level. This lack of guidance results in an inability to function at a political level and, as a consequence of this, to improve patient care. This is based on the premise that poor clinical leadership leads to poor standards of care (Department of Health 1999). There is an urgency, therefore, to address the need for developing leadership skills as an integral aspect of advancing cancer nursing practice.

However, it is not only nurse managers who require leadership skills; for many services the main task of clinical leadership will remain with the charge nurse or their equivalent. Such individuals have a pivotal role in any health service and their leadership is critical to quality care, treatment and outcomes, staff morale and the learning climate of clinical areas (Department of Health 1999). Indeed, the authors of this report contend that these individuals do not always attract the recognition they deserve, yet they remain the backbone of healthcare delivery. The process by which future generations of nurse leaders are identified, nurtured and developed needs first to be defined and then operationalized across Europe.

SECURING AND SUSTAINING A QUALITY CANCER NURSING WORKFORCE

It is frequently acknowledged that there is a direct link between quality service delivery and providing a better quality of working life for staff (NHS Executive 1998). Key service developments in cancer care will succeed only if they are matched with effective planning to ensure a workforce with the necessary capacity, skills and diversity. To enable all nurses engaged in cancer care to contribute fully to the achievement of high-quality service will require the development and nurturing of skills across the entire workforce. Well-managed continuing professional development programmes and innovative approaches to work-based learning and support are also valuable elements in attracting, motivating and retaining high-calibre staff.

The number of nurses worldwide is falling, and recruitment and retention are major concerns in many countries (Salvage & Heijnen 1997). Factors affecting recruitment and retention are complex and interrelated, and the accurate assessment of cause and effect requires a range of demographic, educational and environmental information. Two main issues, however, dominate all discussions: working conditions and the image of nursing (World Health Organization 1996). The history of nursing labour markets is one of a cycle of shortages. Each shortage tends to bring with it a familiar set of proposed solutions: more flexible working hours and the introduction of family-friendly working practices; support for clinical and professional development; career break schemes, etc. Sustained attempts at implementing these solutions, however, have often been lacking. Discussion tends to focus on the general nursing workforce and currently little is understood about recruitment and retention of nursing staff in specialist areas of nursing, including cancer nursing.

The pivotal role of workforce planning, effective personal and organizational development and staff involvement must be recognized to ensure a quality workforce. It is the responsibility of organizations and the individuals within them to meet the challenges confronting cancer care today and to build supportive structures, which deliver quality services and successfully reconcile the needs of staff alongside those of patients. This requires considerable investment, but there is evidence to suggest that such investment, resulting in a cohort of experienced staff, has a direct impact on the outcomes of patient care. Evidence for this statement can be found in the seminal study by Carr-Hill et al (1992). Whilst investigating the links between different skill-mixes and the quality and outcome of care, they concluded that investment in employing qualified staff, providing postqualification training and developing effective methods of organizing care appeared to pay dividends in the delivery of good-quality patient care.

A vision of continuous quality improvement rests on a clear commitment to continuing professional development and lifelong learning by both practitioners and organizations. In planning and providing continuing professional development it should be ensured that it is:

- purposeful and patient centred
- targeted at identified educational need
- educationally effective
- part of any wider organizational development plan in support of local and national service objectives
- focused on the development needs of clinical teams and capable of crossing traditional professional and service boundaries
- designed to build on previous knowledge, skills and experience
- designed to enhance the skills of interpreting and applying knowledge based on research and development.

Nurse managers need to meet local service needs as well as the personal and professional development needs of individuals. Flexible approaches are required to support changing roles and better career pathways, and to foster professional ownership. The learning that takes place at work through experience, critical incidents, audit and reflection, supported by mentorship, clinical supervision and peer review, can be a rich source of learning. Work-based learning in multiprofessional teams, making full use of modern technology, can yield benefits for the individual, the organization and the professions. Often in cancer care settings there are a limited number of nurses, so release of time from clinical responsibilities is limited unless nurses attend on their days off. Flexible and creative educational opportunities need to be developed, capable of responding to such challenges. Nurse managers should be involved in securing suitable continuing education, which reflects the changing patterns of care for patients with cancer. Future trends for cancer care include an increasing elderly population, increasing ethnic diversity, increased reliance on ambulatory and home or community-based cancer care, and treatment focused equally on critical acute episodes and the rehabilitative phases of care.

Any education offered must be accessible, timely, cost effective and fit for purpose. It will be possible to achieve such aspirations for continuing professional development only if nurse managers work strategically with nurse educators within the context of dynamic local forums, thus effectively integrating education and service to enhance nursing care. An integrated approach should successfully match the legitimate aspirations of individual cancer nurses and also respond to local service needs and patient expectations. The risks of relying on the needs perceived by only one group of interested stakeholders should be fully recognized.

There is a lack of empirically based work analysing nurses' perceptions of their continuing professional needs, or the perceived outcomes in terms of changes in knowledge, attitudes, skills, job satisfaction, staff retention and career development (Barriball, While & Norman 1992). Indeed, in an extensive review of the literature by Langton, Blunden & Hek (1999) no research studies were found in which the educational needs of experienced cancer nurses were expressed from this group's perspective. Some evidence as to the perceptions of newly qualified nurses caring for patients with cancer in both general and specialist settings was located, and readers are referred to the full report for details of these.

In the same review referred to above, a lack of reliable studies yielding valid evidence regarding the effectiveness of the delivery of cancer care education and its subsequent impact on the patient experience failed to materialize during the course of the review (Langton, Blunden & Hek 1999). Thus vital information as to what constitutes the most appropriate learning strategies, the contextual features that surround employment, and the specific characteristics of continuing professional development that lead successfully to sustained change in cancer care nursing after any particular programme has ended is conspicuous by its absence. Claims as to the benefits of continuing education are largely anecdotal and much work has yet to be done in refining and applying the evaluative tools that will help in justifying the expense of continuing education in cancer care. Ferguson (1994) does provide some brief examples of work undertaken in this sphere, and Bond & Jodrell (1997) report that nurses who have received new knowledge and skills as a result of education related to cancer care feel empowered and able to make changes to practice. However, very little long-term evaluation of courses has been conducted to identify whether new knowledge and skills are translated into practice and whether patients with cancer are benefiting.

ROLE OF MANAGEMENT IN THE IMPLEMENTATION OF RESEARCH FINDINGS AND QUALITY ASSURANCE

The meaning of theoretical knowledge for professional nursing

Although most nursing scientists see nursing as a practice discipline, the development of theory in nursing presents a means for gaining more recognition as an independent healthcare profession. In healthcare settings that involve a range of other professions, the group holding the theoretical knowledge that relates to a specific issue is the most likely to provide effective therapy. This issue will then become the domain of that particular profession (Ingram 1991). Whilst the pursuit of power cannot be justified as an end in itself, the contribution of nursing to healthcare can become significant if it achieves professional autonomy. Nursing theory as a source of professional autonomy will provide a solid base for challenging existing healthcare practice. Furthermore, new analytical skills will help nurse scientists to act deliberately. Because nursing is a science-based, practical discipline, the quote by Fawcett (1980, p. 10) may be very relevant for its future:

A theory in and of itself is irrelevant – and a practice devoid of theoretically sound, empirically validated processes may soon be considered as unethical.

If theory is considered the foundation of nursing practice, academically trained nurses in leadership positions in nursing practice, education and research will have a profound impact on the future of nursing. However, it is a challenge to overcome the, often blamed, practice–theory gap. Nursing will build up its scientific knowledge only if it represents a logically connected network of theories that represent the current view concerning the natural world of nursing (Crow 1982).

More and more nurses in Europe now have the opportunity to experience the transition from diploma to doctoral nurse. A deeper understanding of nursing and caring can be expected. Theory, therefore, does not necessarily alienate nursing from caring; it can make nursing more interesting and precious. Undoubtedly, academic nurses still have to convince many nursing colleagues, and also physicians and the public, about the necessity of a theoretical foundation. Moreover, it has been cautioned that the route of science alone is a dangerous one for nursing. It can be argued that the development of science can also contribute to the development of a practice-based, nurturing role for nursing. This very special role in caring for a vulnerable person and their family includes the message 'we are there for you'. Yet, we remain united as a profession to communicate this central image of nursing to the public and the interdisciplinary team. Kitson (1996) has argued that tensions within our profession inhibit that image: tensions between the autonomous practitioner versus the subservient employee, tensions around the contemporary strategy of promoting advanced practitioners which can induce negative feelings in the majority of nurses, who are not, never will be, and even do not need to be advanced practitioners. However, if science can show the majority of nurses how precious their caring, nurturing role is and how it might influence effective care, science fulfils the role of defining caring as a human mode of being (Roach 1984). During the last decade, nurses had problems in accepting the fact that helping and assisting are integral elements of nursing. 'Being there for you', however, is not a message of submissiveness, it rather is a message of skilled companionship and human being. It appears that, these days, we need to relearn what care really means. Nursing concepts and theories that perfectly conceptualize this notion of 'being there for you' (Gaut 1983, Griffin 1983) were described some time ago.

Implementing research into practice: overcoming the practice–theory gap

Nursing scientists are able to develop evidence-based nursing practice, establish nursing research units and academic programmes. However, pursuing an elitist nursing agenda carries the danger of alienating the majority of nurses at the bedside because nurses from most countries are not academically trained. If the vision of evidence-based practice and nursing as a science-based discipline is to become reality, the impact of the so-called 'knowledge generators' has to improve. There seems to be a hierarchical split between those who do research and those who should use research results. The knowledge generators, usually researchers, lecturers and other academics, 'hand down' their research findings, theories and models to practising nursing colleagues who are then expected to understand and implement them in clinical areas.

This attitude of scientists towards practitioners might be part of the 'practice–theory gap', which poses a serious problem for the further development of the nursing profession. This does not mean that the available research is inappropriate, but it means that there is a communication problem within the different disciplines of nursing. Gibbings (1993, p. 30) has made it explicit in that:

> ... the blame for the continuation of traditional practices, which research has shown should be changed, cannot be laid at the door of that research. Rather the fault is either one of communication of findings, or of inertia to change.

A problem that might contribute to this can be seen in the professional positions of nursing scientists. Whilst medical colleagues do research as part of patient care, nurse scientists rarely have a position directly involved with patient care. Can nurse scientists in the so-called 'ivory towers' of universities and schools prioritize research needs? Nurses at the bedside often cannot understand the amount of effort used to do research in relation to models and theories, which have little influence on apparently existing practical problems. A further problem has been suggested by Hall (1986), who states that nurses, as a response to that alienation, become more psychologically minded and that physical care, which is still a very substantial part of nursing practice, remains neglected or is seen as second best. Kitson (1996) describes this tendency as 'selling out the caring birthright for a mess of psychological pottage' (p. 1649). Research activities need to be prioritized according to the needs of patients and it has to be carried out in collaboration with practising colleagues. Theorists, who are out of touch with the needs and realities of clinical practice, might end up with irrelevant research questions, and likewise with irrelevant answers.

The theory–practice gap, however, has two sides. Practitioners, who should be the 'knowledge appliers', have problems in turning results into research-based practice (Hunt 1996), either by not being aware of current research findings or by not implementing them properly. Apart from the above-mentioned communication problem, nurses might not be prepared to think in a research-minded manner and therefore prefer to feel secure with traditional routines. This phenomenon may be observed in nurses at the bedside but also in nurse managers (Rutledge et al 1998). Traditional routines, however, will not be successful strategies through which to change the environment, and nurse managers will have to tackle this problem if the profession is to survive the new millennium.

One solution to closing the practice–theory gap has been described where the practitioner becomes directly involved in nursing research rather than relying on academics. Action research methodologies have been used for such practice-based nursing projects (Hart 1996). Even though this sounds promising, we need to be cautious in producing knowledge that might not fulfil the full criteria of science. Practitioners who want to do research in the practical field should not hesitate to enter into collaboration with those who have knowledge of research methods. Science without the personal and practical involvement of scientists cannot serve the image of the nursing profession. Nurse leaders should be challenged but not frightened to communicate with scientists. Here, it becomes evident again that nurse managers need to be strong leaders who do not act to limit choices but are open to develop fresh approaches to long-standing problems (Zaleznik 1977). If nurse managers do not support the bringing about of change, research findings will not be adopted in clinical practice.

Management of change: the basis for evidence-based practice and quality assurance

Implementing research-based practice is closely linked to overcoming inertia to change. This is an essential challenge to nurse managers. Planned change is a complex process, a conscious, deliberate and collaborative effort to improve operations of human systems through utilization of valid knowledge (Bennis, Benne & Chin 1985). The target of change can be the person's knowledge, the person's attitude or the person's or even a group's behaviour. Whilst a change in knowledge may occur with little difficulty and in a short time period, a change in behaviour will be much more difficult and involve a longer time period (Hersey & Blanchard 1988). The most difficult change involves a change in behaviour in a group, which is often the case if changes in nursing practice have to be implemented. The person appointed to be in charge of the change process needs to be selected carefully, as the sanction and support of the group can be extremely important in the change process (Kemp 1984). The driving forces, such as motivation, and the restraining forces, such as anxiety and the wish to maintain the status quo, need attention, support and guidance. Change will be adopted only if it is rationally justified and if some gain can be recognized (Bernhard & Walsh 1990).

In order to implement evidence-based practice, nurse managers require two crucial competencies: to be informed about new scientific evidence in nursing and to be able to prepare and support the process of change in an institution. Research, unfortunately, has shown that practitioners have many reasons for not implementing research in practice, one of which is not being allowed to do so by their leaders (Hunt 1996). This means that nursing managers must hold the expressed aim of developing nursing within the framework of leadership. Leadership has been defined as a process that is used to move a group towards goal-setting and attainment, which is an essential component in nursing (Bernhard & Walsh 1990). Essential characteristics of leadership have been defined by Shaw (1989) as 'having a clear vision of the future, visibility (leaders take people with them), being a risk taker and one who permits and encourages risk-taking in others, a generator of enthusiasm and motivation to shared goals and values, commitment and sense of purpose'. Shaw (1989) emphasized the importance of charismatic leadership qualities, but it has also been concluded that individuals who are selected for management positions need special (managerial) preparation and personal characteristics (Lorentzon 1992). It could be concluded that a nurse leader in the field of practice, education and research needs to be both an enthusiastic nurse and a leader with interpersonal skills, preferably with a scientific background, in order to support and implement evidence-based practice.

Quality assurance: a continuous challenge for nurse managers

Quality assurance is a continuously challenging process and, for the process to be successful, nurse leaders and staff nurses need to overcome inertia to change. As some domains of nursing activity are difficult to assess and measure, nurses tend to dismiss ways of setting standards and processes surrounding quality assurance. A future with increasing pressure on nurses to be more accurate is likely with the development of Total Quality Management. If nurses want to be accountable for their practice, they need to pay attention to its regulation. If they fail to do so, there is danger that others, such as political or institutional authorities, will do it for them. One major concern for nurses is the fear of losing creativity and becoming severely restricted with respect to practice (Schmidli 1995). Whilst such fear is not unsubstantiated, it can be argued that standards of care must be a dynamic instrument, where changes can be discussed and agreed with the persons in charge. On the other hand, it cannot be denied that adherence to care standards aims to prevent poor quality, which is the ultimate aim of quality assurance.

Quality management translates into taking a leading role in the politics of quality within an institution, which includes the setting of general objectives, supporting their finance, and facilitating planning, measuring, evaluating and improving quality of care (Gehrig 1995). Whilst a professional association or a hospital sets universal objectives for care, the clinical nurse manager is in a unique position to influence quality assurance at the local level (Oroviogoicoechea 1996). The effectiveness of this role is based on the fact that it represents a link between management and employees, and is thus positioned in the locations where care and quality assurance is facilitated. The American Organization of Nurse Executives (AONE 1992, p. 36) has formulated the following definition:

The nurse manager is central to effective, quality patient care. The nurse manager has become a more visible position within the health care institution, serving as a vital link between the larger vision of health care institution and the unit based delivery of effective, high quality patient care.

Quality of care can be seen from different viewpoints, one of which is reflected in political decisions which might be made that are beyond the major influence of individual professionals. If healthcare restructuring efforts are guided more by costs than by quality, this will have a profound impact on quality patient care. Such developments, including restricted access to specialized oncology care, imposing limitations on treatment selection, and the dissolution of specialized oncology units, have been observed by the American Oncology Nursing Society. This society felt strongly enough on this issue to compose a position paper on Quality Cancer Care (Mooney 1997). European countries will not be isolated from such worrying developments.

Nurse managers should facilitate standard-setting within given possibilities and limits. This means that quality must be defined on the basis of available resources. The definition of quality pays regard to this: 'quality is an agreed level of excellence' (Donabedian 1988, p. 132). Quality assurance means assuring the consumer of nursing a specified degree of excellence through measurement and evaluation (Schmadl 1979).

Consumers of nursing care, however, might not really know what kind of care they can expect, and are mostly unable to make comparisons. Patient satisfaction with care is often evaluated by asking recipients of care to fill in a postcare questionnaire. Even though this is a widely used method in assessing quality, it might be difficult for some patients to be honest because they fear that they might be in need of the service in future. Still, asking patients and relatives about the performance of activities (not about the performer) seems an indispensable approach in relation to the evaluation of care. Quality assurance generally includes the following elements (Pearson 1992):

- setting objectives and standard criteria (reflecting the agreed level of quality and the way to achieve it)
- evaluation of standardized care through measurement
- acting on the evaluation.

Different quality and audit systems have been implemented to assure quality in nursing care. Instruments such as peer reviews (Pearson 1992), the Quality of Patient Care Scale (Wandelt & Ager 1974), Phaneuf's Audit (Phaneuf 1976) and Monitor (Goldstone, Ball & Collier 1983) are some of the currently well-used methods. For a description of these methods the reader is referred to the specific literature (Sale 1990). One major concern is the fact that, as yet, there is little evidence to suggest that they are having any significant impact in terms of changing practice and improving patient care (Harvey & Kitson 1996). It has been concluded that the integration of clinical audit into the quality management structures of an organization as a whole requires facilitators (such as managers) who take on the vital role of catalyst and change agent, and as promoter of necessary coordination, networking and support of quality improvement strategies (Harvey & Kitson 1996).

One of the key issues in quality assurance is the question of who is going to set standards and evaluate quality. The subjective nature of nursing is connected to that of values, attitudes and opinion, which make up professional judgement. Nurses in practice, education or management are therefore the logical source of standard statements, provided they seek validation of their ideas from those who are involved in the activity and from those who hold the scientific knowledge. Nursing leadership in quality assurance therefore means to encourage meaningful participation in the quality programme and giving staff a sense of control over its direction. This includes much more than simply providing staff with information. This aspect has been mentioned in association with the term 'ownership for quality' and it has been shown that this is the level of responsibility and involvement that clinical staff want to take on board (Harvey & Kitson 1996). 'Ownership for quality' has been said to be promoted more rapidly through bottom-up approaches to implementation rather than a top-down strategy (Harvey & Kitson 1996). Consideration of the leadership style of nurse managers appears to be particularly relevant in implementing a quality assurance programme.

Steps in the implementation of a quality assurance programme – an example from Switzerland

Universal standards concern the philosophy and ethics of the profession and are rather abstract, usually developed by nurses' associations or healthcare authorities. Universal standards of nursing care in cancer care have, for example, been edited by the Royal College of Nursing (1991). Universal standards are difficult to measure directly but represent foundations through which to build further, more specific, standards. An institution will formulate standards that represent expectations and general objectives for the whole institution. Finally, local standards describe standards with measurable criteria within a ward or other working unit (Sale 1990).

A quality assurance programme with institutional and local care standards was implemented in a teaching hospital in St Gallen, Switzerland. The implementation of this project will be summarized here. In 1993 the local government ordered the implementation of quality assurance programmes in healthcare. Prior to implementation, the nursing director had engaged a small group of nurse managers and educators to redefine a philosophy of care for the hospital. Following that, a core group of nursing experts, again from the educational and management departments, was created in order to formulate universal, institutional standards of care for the hospital.

After agreement was reached on these institutional standards by all nurse managers, it was decided that in order to produce the local standards a bottom-up approach should be used. Educational workshops were provided for staff nurses about quality assurance in general, and the development of nursing standards specifically, using the structure, process and outcome criteria described by Donabedian (1988). The activity of setting standards and describing related measurement criteria were delegated to the level at which they would be implemented, practised and evaluated. As a standard presents the level that others accept as the baseline for good practice (Pearson 1992), this bottom-up approach was expected to favour ownership of quality at the ward level.

Staff nurses were enthusiastic about their ability to set standards for their 'real world' and to demonstrate accountability in their work. Setting standards is a difficult task, so the staff nurses were supported by one of the nurse experts belonging to the core expert group. Most needed specific support in producing the texts. When a standard was written, the nurse expert from the core team confirmed that it was not contradictory to the hospital standards, that it had a scientific rational (where applicable) and that the criteria were measurable and coherent in relation to structure, process and outcome. If it fulfilled these criteria, it had to be signed by those who set the standards, the head nurse, other disciplines involved and the expert nurse. Implementation of the standard first took place within the team with which it was produced, but was often soon adopted by other teams in the same department, sometimes with few changes.

Meanwhile, a group of experienced clinical staff nurses were trained as members of a quality measurement group, using the peer review method. This method is defined as a process by which practitioners of the same rank, profession or setting critically appraise one another's work performance against established standards (O'Laughlin & Kaulbach 1981). This method has the advantage that results carry more credibility, evaluation provides insight into shortcomings of own practice and required changes are more likely to occur (Pearson 1992).

Self-evaluation within the ward was practised twice a year. This gave an opportunity to check the adoption of standards by the team members. One year after implementation of the quality assurance programme, the specially prepared peers from the quality measurement group, not working within the ward where the evaluation took place, started to measure and evaluate standards on an annual basis. Measuring included the evaluation of specific standard criteria by observation of structure and process on the ward, asking the nurses involved (especially as concerns process), consulting members of other disciplines if applicable, enlisting opinions of patients concerning specific nursing activities, and reading the nursing documentation. The reviewers documented their review findings on specially prepared forms. The report was then presented to the ward sister and the head nurse in order to set new objectives and plan courses of action.

Finally, the head nurse was required to support the ward sister in taking action, if needed, and to monitor the whole assurance process. As the strategy 'management by objectives' was already implemented in the hospital, contracting was used as a helpful technique to guide any course of action.

This example shows that a quality assurance process can be implemented if a clear management plan allows for facilitation and support for development of knowledge, activities and attitudes in the field. The amount of commitment, time and money needed to maintain a continuing quality assurance process should not, however, be underestimated. Quality has its price and it cannot be assured through the voluntary work of nurses. On the other hand, it is well known that poor quality can be much more expensive than good quality. Furthermore, for professional nurses who strive for reflective, evidence-based practice, the quality assurance process might present a precious instrument through which to achieve their goals.

INTEGRATED CARE PATHWAYS

Another means of ensuring the delivery of quality care may be a move towards pathways of care. It has been argued that managed care programmes can promote the delivery of a quality service (Ellis 1997). The term 'managed care' is being developed across Europe following its conception in the USA. Managing care effectively involves the provision of a controlled environment that delivers effective care, taking account of the potential risks and control of inappropriate costs (Johnson 1997). One way of achieving this is through the use of clinical care pathways. Such pathways can facilitate a collaborative multiprofessional approach to care. Probably the best known example of a managed care programme is the integrated care pathway (ICP).

ICP is simply a tool that enables the identification of a specific client group and delineation of a care pathway of anticipated care. Ideally, this should be done from a multidisciplinary perspective, thereby ensuring a comprehensive approach to patient care. Adopting the ICP ensures a consistent approach to management for similar groups of patients. When the pathway is implemented, all those involved with the care of the patient follow the care as directed by the pathway and any variance to care is noted. Analysis of the variance provides data on actual care compared with the anticipated care identified in the pathway, resulting in an ongoing clinical audit of practice (Johnson 1997). It has been argued that the use of ICPs has led to reductions in lengths of stay (Buchanan & Smith 1993, Campedelli 1994, Johnson 1995), reductions in cost (Morris & Mylotte 1995), and improved patient satisfaction and clinical outcome (Morris & Welsh 1996). However, these claims are largely anecdotal and to date there is little scientific research to support them (Johnson 1997).

Notwithstanding the lack of empirical evidence as to the value of ICPs, it is beyond doubt that an integrated approach to care which is systematic in its approach is much needed in healthcare, particularly in this era of cost containment. Adopting a pathway of care model in cancer care would harness the multiprofessional approach to care that is acclaimed rhetorically but in reality seldom practised. In many situations it is nurses who are leading the shift towards integrated care providing, it is argued, real benefits to patients, effective multidisciplinary team-working and the promotion of evidence-based practice. The pathways in cancer care prepared by North West Nurses and Professions Allied to Medicine Cancer Services Steering Group (1998) build on current and emerging practice and depict a scheme for representing the journey undertaken by individual patients, their families and carers. Such pathways, when constructed rigorously, facilitate nurses in articulating clearly how they, as a professional group, plan and manage care, the complementary roles of both specialist and generic nurses, and the criteria against which care might be evaluated.

Another example of the shift away from the biomedical approach to care is the emergence of nurse-led services in a number of areas, including breast cancer (Earnshaw & Stephenson 1997), breathlessness (Bredin et al 1999), brain tumours (James, Guerrero & Brada 1994) and prostate cancer (Faithful 1999). Through the reorientation of healthcare services, patients are being afforded a more individual service which better addresses their comprehensive needs whilst maintaining the follow-up that is necessary in relation to disease management.

CONCLUSION

If nurses are to continue to influence the delivery of cancer care, several factors are critical. Uppermost is the concept of leadership, which is a key skill of any cancer nurse practising at an advanced level. Following from this, a sound knowledge platform of management strategies to ensure an appropriate nurse workforce should facilitate optimal patient care. As yet, however, we are far from this reality in Europe, and as a consequence we have a responsibility to continue to strive towards the attainment of a European specialty of cancer nursing. Such recognition would enable the potential of cancer nursing to be realized. In our efforts to attain this recognition, we should remember the strength to be gained by working in collaboration with all colleagues in cancer care to ensure that nursing is an equal partner in care management.

REFERENCES

Alexander D 1993 Staff support groups: do they support and are they even groups? Palliative Medicine 7:127–132

American Organization of Nurse Executives 1992 The role and functions of the nurse manager. Nursing Management 23(9):36–38

Astudillo W, Mendinueta C 1996 Exhaustion syndrome in palliative care. Supportive Care Cancer 4:408–415

Australian Institute of Health and Welfare 1994 Health Expenditure Bulletin No 10, December 1994

Barriball K, While A, Norman I 1992 Continuing professional education for qualified nurses: a review of the literature. Journal of Advanced Nursing 17:1129–1140

Benner P, Wrubel J 1989 The primacy of caring. Menlo Park, California, Addison-Weseley

Bennis W, Nanus B 1985 Leaders: the strategies for taking charge. Harper and Row, New York

Bennis W, Benne K, Chin R 1985 The planning of change, 4th edn. Holt Reinhart & Winston, New York

Bernard B, Walsh M 1990 Leadership: the key to the professionalisation of nursing, 2nd edn. Mosby, St Louis

Bond P, Jodrell N 1997 Cancer nursing in Europe: an account based on interviews with students, nurses and doctors. Journal of Cancer Nursing 1(2):81–85

Bredin M, Corner J, Krishnasamy M, Plant H, Bailey C, A'Hern R 1999 Multicentre randomised controlled trial of nursing intervention for breathlessness in patients with lung cancer. British Medical Journal 318(7188):901

Buchanan L, Smith J 1993 Pathway to recovery: using anticipated recovery pathways. Healthcare Today Spring:20–21

Busch R, McMillan S 1993 Validity and reliability of a bone marrow transplant acuity tool. Oncology Nursing Forum 20(9):1385–1392

Busch R, Reardon M, Gordon B, McMillan S 1994 Validity and reliability of medical and surgical oncology patient acuity tools. Oncology Nursing Forum 21 (10):1709–1717

Campbell A 1984 Nursing, nurturing and sexism. In: Campbell A (ed) Moderated love: a theology of professional care. SPCK, London

Campedelli B 1994 Integrated care pathways. NHS Executive VFM Update, II, London

Carr-Hill R, Dixon P, Gibbs I et al 1992 Skill mix and the effectiveness of nursing care. Centre for Health Economics, University of York, York

Crow R 1982 Frontiers of nursing in the twenty-first century: development of models and theories on the concept of nursing. Journal of Advanced Nursing 7:111–116

Dean M 1992 Nursing's identity crisis. Lancet 339:1160–1161

Department of Health 1999 Making a difference. Strengthening the nursing, midwifery and health visiting contribution to health and healthcare. Department of Health, London

Donabedian A 1988 Quality assessment and assurance: unity of purpose, diversity and means. Inquiry 25:173–192

Earnshaw J, Stephenson Y 1997 First two years of a follow up breast clinic led by a nurse practitioner. Journal of the Royal Society of Medicine 90:258–259

Ellis B W 1997 Managed care: a hospital clinician's view. Journal of Managed Care 1:9–11

Faithful S 1999 Randomised trial, a method of comparisons: a study of supportive care in radiotherapy nursing. European Oncology Nursing Journal 3(3):176–184

Fawcett J 1980 A framework for analysis and evaluation of conceptual models of nursing. Nurse Educator 5(6):10–14

Ferguson A 1994 Evaluating the purpose and benefits of continuing education in nursing and the implications for the provision of continuing education for cancer nurses. Journal of Advanced Nursing 19:640–646

Gaut D 1983 Development of a theoretically adequate description of caring. Western Journal of Nursing Research 5(4):313–324

Gehrig O 1995 Einige Elemente zum Thema Qualitätsmanagement. Schweizer Spital 4:18–19

Gibbings S 1993 Informed action. Nursing Times 89(46):28–31

Goldstone L A, Ball J, Collier M 1983 Monitor: an index of the quality of nursing care for acute medical and surgical wards. Newcastle upon Tyne Polytechnic Products, Newcastle upon Tyne

Griffin A 1983 A philosophical analysis of care in nursing. Journal of Advanced Nursing 8:289–295

Hall L 1986 Another view of nursing care and quality. In: Straub K (ed) Continuity of patient care; the role of nursing. Catholic University Press, Washington, DC, p 47

Halloran E 1983 'RN staffing – more care – less cost'. Nurse Management 14(9):18–22

Hart E 1996 Action research as a professionalising strategy: issues and dilemmas. Journal of Advanced Nursing 23:454–461

Harvey G, Kitson A 1996 Achieving improvement through quality: an evaluation of key factors in the implementation process. Journal of Advanced Nursing 24:185–195

Hendricks J 1997 The pricing of nursing care. Journal of Advanced Nursing 25:454–462

Hersey P, Blanchard K 1988 Management of organisational behaviour: utilisation of human resources, 5th edn. Prentice-Hall, Englewood Cliffs, New Jersey

Hoffman M L 1981 Is altruism part of human nature? Journal of Personality and Social Psychology 40:121–137

Hunt J 1996 Barriers to research utilization. Journal of Advanced Nursing 23:423–425 (Editorial)

Ingram R 1991 Why does nursing need theory? Journal of Advanced Nursing 16:350–353

James N, Guerrero D, Brada M 1994 Who should follow up cancer patients? Nurse specialist based outpatient care and the introduction a phone clinic system. Clinical Oncology 6(5):283–287

Johnson S 1995 Pathway to the heart of quality. Nursing Management 8(1):26–27

Johnson S 1997 Pathways of care: what and how? Journal of Managed Care 1:15–17

King's Fund Management College 1995 Johnson and Johnson/King's Fund Nursing Leadership Programme. Needs assessment. King's Fund, London

Kemp V 1984 An overview of change and leadership. Topics in Clinical Nursing 6(1):1–9

Kitson A 1996 Does nursing have a future? British Medical Journal 313:1647–1651

Kuhn B 1980 Prediction of nursing requirements from patient characteristics. International Journal Nursing Studies 17:5–15

Langton H, Blunden G, Hek G 1999 Cancer nursing literature review and documentary analysis. English National Board for Nursing, Midwifery and Health Visiting, London

Lees S 1990 The design of a stress management programme for nursing personnel. Journal of Advanced Nursing 15:946–961

Lorentzon M 1992 Authority, leadership and management in nursing. Journal of Advanced Nursing 17:525–527 (Editorial)

Lovett R, Wagner L, McMillan S 1991 Validity and reliability of a pediatric hematology oncology patient acuity tool. Journal of Pediatric Oncology Nursing 8(3):122–130

Mäder C, Bamert U 1994 Pflegeaufwand Mess-System PAMS. Ein Handbuch für die Leistungserfassung in der Krankenpflege im Akutspital. LEP Sekretariat, Kantonsspital, 9007 St Gallen, Switzerland

Magnusson L 1985 The development and validation of an oncology patient classification system. Oncology Nursing Forum 12(6):17–22

Marsee V, Busch R, McMillan S 1995 Validity and reliability of an oncology critical care patient tool. Oncology Nursing Forum 22(6):967–971

Maslach C 1982 Burnout – a review of the literature with application to cancer nursing. Cancer Nursing 2:211–217

Mayrhofer M 1997 Leistungserfassung mit LEP: Ein Managementinstrument für die Pflege. Schweizer Spital 8:26–27

Meyers D 1985 The GRASP system. Journal of Nursing Administration 15(12):2

Mooney C 1997 Oncology nursing position paper on quality of cancer care. Oncology Nursing Forum 24(6):951–953

Morris E, Mylotte A 1995 The management of childhood asthma through care pathways. Nursing Times 46(91):36–37

Morris E, Welsh R 1996 Heart to heart. Health Service Journal 3:33

North West Nurses & Professions Allied to Medicine Cancer Services Steering Group (1998) Pathways in cancer care. NHS Executive North West, Department of Health, Warrington, UK

O'Laughlin E, Kaulbach D 1981 Peer review: a model for performance appraisal. Journal of Nursing Administration September:22–27

Oroviogoicoechea C 1996 The clinical nurse manager: a literature review. Journal of Advanced Nursing 24:1273–1280

NHS Executive 1998 Working together. Securing a quality workforce for the NHS. Department of Health, Leeds

Pearson A 1992 Nursing quality measurement. John Wiley, Chichester, UK

Pfefferkorn B, Rovetta C 1940 Administrative cost analysis for nursing service and education. American Hospital Association and National League of Nursing Education, Chicago

Phaneuf M C 1976 The nursing audit: self regulation in nursing practice. Appleton-Century-Crofts, New York

Reid N, Melaugh M 1987 Nurse hours per patient: a method for monitoring and explaining staffing levels. International Journal of Nursing Studies 24(1):1–14

Roach S 1984 The human mode of being: implications for nursing. Faculty of Nursing, University of Toronto, Toronto

Royal College of Nursing 1991 Standards of care. Cancer nursing. Scutari Projects, Harrow, UK

Rutledge D, Ropka M, Green P, Nail N, Mooney K 1998 Barriers to research utilization for oncology staff nurses and nurse managers/clinical nurse specialists. Oncology Nursing Forum 25(3):497–506

Sale D 1990 Quality assurance: essentials of nursing management. Macmillan, London

Salvage J, Heijnen S 1997 Nursing in Europe. A resource for better health. European Series No 74. World Health Organization Regional Publications, Geneva

Scher B 1988 'Are checklists replacing good care?' Nursing January (1):47

Schmadl J 1979 Quality assurance: examination of the concept. Nursing Outlook 27(7):462–465

Schmidli C 1995 Qualitätssicherung in der Pflege an einem Kantonsspital. Pflege 8(4):324–332

Shaw S 1989 Nurses in management: new challenges, new opportunities. International Nursing Review 36(6):179–184

Stefan S, Gillies D A, Biordi S 1992 Nursing care costs for a DRG sub group. Nursing Economics 10(4):277–280

Tannenbaum R, Weschler IR, Massarik F 1974 Leadership: a frame of reference. In: Cathcart RS, Samopvar LA (eds). Small group communication: a reader. William C Brown, Dubuque

Tappen R 1989 Nursing leadership and management: concepts and practice. F A Davis, Philadelphia

Thibault C, David N, O'Brian L, Vinet A 1990 Workload measurment systems in nursing. Association des hopitaux du Quebec, National Library of Canada, Quebec

Ullrich A 1990 Stress experienced by physicians and nurses in the cancer ward. Oxford University Press, Oxford

Van Dam F 1990 A 14 year investigation into the workload of oncology nurses in the Netherlands Cancer Institute. Cancer Nursing 13(6):17–22

Wandelt M A, Ager J W 1974 Quality patient care scale. Appleton-Century-Crofts, New York

World Health Organization 1996 Nursing practice. Report of a WHO expert committee. WHO Technical Report Series No 860. WHO, Geneva

Yasko J, Fleck A 1984 Prospective payment (DRG): what will be the impact on cancer care? Oncology Nursing Forum 11(3):69

Zaleznik A 1977 Managers and leaders: are they different? Harvard Business Review May–June:67–78

Clinical decision-making

Kathy Redmond

CHAPTER

4

INTRODUCTION

Every day nurses are called upon to make clinical judgements, for which they are both responsible and accountable. Clinical decision-making is a complex and uncertain process, not least because of the large number of factors that influence a nurse's ability to arrive at an optimal clinical judgement. There is no one theory of decision-making in nursing; indeed, the literature on this subject is awash with conflicting philosophies and definitions, which has resulted in an enormous lack of clarity. Furthermore, there is no clear consensus about the usefulness or validity of approaches to clinical decision-making such as the nursing process and nursing diagnosis.

The purpose of this chapter is to clarify what is meant by clinical decision-making and to explore how nurses go about making judgements in everyday clinical practice. It is important to note that the literature on clinical decision-making is generic to all nursing specialties. However, there is a dearth of research on clinical decision-making in cancer nursing and, indeed, in nursing *per se*. This makes it impossible to produce a research-based chapter on clinical decision-making in cancer nursing without extrapolating results from studies on this subject carried out on other nursing specialties and in medicine. To help readers apply some of the theoretical and practical aspects of clinical decision-making to cancer nursing, a number of examples that relate to the specialty are included.

THE NATURE OF CLINICAL DECISION-MAKING

A definition of clinical judgement, clinical decision-making and problem-solving

A brief perusal of the literature on clinical decision-making in nursing will reveal that the terms clinical decision-making, clinical judgement and problem-solving are often used interchangeably, although not in a distinct manner. These terms are linked, but they do not mean the same thing, and clearly some effort is required to define them in order to clarify their meaning. This is difficult since the terms are vague and ambiguous in that several possible meanings may apply. However, Chinn & Jacob (1983) maintain that ambiguities exist in all definitions, hence, defining terms often requires reconciliation of different and often competing meanings. The rules governing the use of a word are the rules that define that word (Bandman & Bandman 1995). This means that when a precise set of rules for using a word is absent, reasonable definitions are neither right nor wrong. Thus, in order to arrive at a useful definition, one should identify the different meanings that apply to a term, examine them for commonalities and differences, and then decide which of the meanings best clarifies the term as it applies to nursing. What follows, therefore, is an exploration of the terms clinical decision-making, clinical judgement and problem-solving, with the purpose of establishing a stipulative definition for each term. A stipulative definition states how an individual intends to use a term in a given context (Bandman & Bandman 1995).

Judgement, decision-making and problem-solving have been defined by numerous authors, and some examples are offered in Box 4.1. Some authors have defined judgement in terms of a process that involves a series of decisions (Carnevali & Durand Thomas 1993, Pellegrino 1979, Tanner 1987), whereas others have defined it in terms of a statement of a condition that is made as a result of a decision-making process (Yates 1990). Similarly, Carroll & Johnson (1990) have stated that judgement is a kind of decision task where a label is placed on a single alternative or attribute. For example, one may judge that a person is anxious or in pain, or that

---

■ **BOX 4.1   A selection of definitions of judgement, decision-making and problem-solving**

Judgement

'A multi-step, end-orientated concatenation of decisions demanding different types of reasons and reasoning which will justify a particular course of action, for a particular patient, given that patient's particular existential situation at the time of the decision' (Pellegrino 1979, p. 170).

'The evaluation of one or more possibilities with respect to a specific set of evidence and goals' (Baron 1988, p. 6).

'A statement which expresses the condition or situation' or 'a statement which expresses the condition or situation as an evaluation such as a quantitative analogy (e.g. the condition is better than before)' (Yates 1990, cited by Crow, Chase & Lamond 1995, p. 207).

'The series of decisions made by the nurse in interaction with the client regarding (a) the type of observation to be made in the client situation, (b) the evaluation of the data observed and the derivation of meaning (diagnosis), (c) nursing actions that should be taken with or on behalf of the client (management)' (Tanner 1987, p. 154).

'Judgement and choice are two different kinds of decision making that can, at times, produce different decisions' (Carroll & Johnson 1990, p. 23).

'Clinical judgements are complex decisions about the status of an individual or family and the contextual situation affecting the person's or family's responses based on findings and their interpretation' (Carnevali & Durand Thomas 1993, p. 3).

'The ways in which nurses come to understand the problems, issues or concerns of patients, to attend to salient information, and to respond in concerned and involved ways' (Tanner 1993, p. 17).

Decision-making

'An act of selecting a choice among two or more possible alternatives for a prospective action' (Kim 1983, p. 276).

'A decision is a choice of action – of what to do or not to do' (Baron 1988, p. 3).

'A choice is made among a number of possible alternatives, often involving trade-offs among the values given to different outcomes' (Baumann & Deber 1989, p. 1).

'A process by which a person, group, or organization identifies a choice or judgement to be made, gathers and evaluates information about alternatives, and selects from among the alternatives' (Carroll & Johnson 1990, p. 19).

Problem-solving

'The search for a correct solution to a problem ... the process (problem solving) resembles the orderly steps of decision making, but tends to assume that one correct answer is being sought' (Baumann & Deber 1989, p. 1).

they require a particular intervention. Carroll & Johnson (1990) differentiate a judgement task from a choice task and propose that a choice involves making comparisons among alternatives. In contrast, Baron (1988) views judgement as an evaluation of one or more possibilities. This corresponds with Carroll & Johnson's (1990) definition of a choice as opposed to a judgement task. Tanner (1987, 1993) has proposed two distinctly different definitions of judgement. Her first indicates that judgement involves a series of decisions, whereas her second definition is much broader and does not refer to decision-making. One could argue, however, that when Tanner (1993) uses the term 'ways' she is actually referring to a series of decisions.

In summary, then, judgement is defined both as a process of decision-making and as an outcome of that process. Neither of these meanings is incorrect; however, for the purpose of this chapter judgement is defined as the choice that is made at the end of a decision-making process (i.e. what is actually decided).

Decision-making is more clearly defined in the literature in that it seems to involve making a choice between a number of different alternatives. The decision could well be that nothing is wrong or that no intervention is required. In contrast, problem-solving is about finding solutions to problems. By definition, then, a problem must exist before it can be solved. Moreover, the problem-solving process will incorporate decision-making in that choices need to be made about what is wrong and what is the best way to solve the problem. The assumption in Baumann & Deber's (1989) definition of problem-solving, that there is one correct answer to a problem, is appropriate for some problems, such as those in mathematics and the natural sciences; however, the applicability of this definition to the types of complex problems nurses and doctors confront in clinical practice could be questioned. The steps of the decision and problem-solving process have been

---

■ **BOX 4.2   Difference between the stages of the problem-solving and decision-making process**

Problem-solving

- Assessment
  - problem recognition
  - data-gathering and analysis.
- Diagnosis
  - decide what is wrong
  - decide prognosis.
- Planning
  - goal-setting
  - decide on treatment.
- Implementation
  - carry out plan.
- Evaluation
  - consider response to intervention.

Source: Baumann & Deber (1989),
Carnevali & Durand Thomas (1993)

Decision-making

- Recognition
  - realize that there is a decision to make.
- Formulation
  - explore and classify the decision situation.
- Alternative generation
  - identify all possible alternatives.
- Information search
  - identify the attributes and properties of alternatives under consideration.
- Judgement or choice
  - place a label on a single alternative (judgement)
  - make comparison among alternatives (choice).
- Action and feedback
  - act upon decision
  - consider outcome of the action.

Source: Carroll & Johnson (1990)

> ■ **BOX 4.3** **Stipulative definitions of judgement, decision-making and problem-solving**
>
> A *judgement* is the choice that is made at the end of a decision-making process.
>
> *Decision-making* is a cognitive process that involves making a choice between a number of different alternatives in order to arrive at a judgement.
>
> *Problem-solving* is a cognitive process where judgements are made in order to arrive at a correct or optimal solution to a particular problem.

outlined in Box 4.2, and this may help readers to see the close link between the two concepts, but also highlight their differences.

In conclusion, decision-making is about making a choice between different alternatives. The choice may be that a problem does not exist, that the patient is not at risk or that no intervention is required. On the other hand, problem-solving is a cognitive process whereby judgements are made in order to arrive at a correct or optimal solution to a particular problem (Box 4.3).

THE SCOPE OF DECISION-MAKING IN NURSING

Nurses make a range of different judgements in their everyday clinical practice. According to Tanner (1987), nursing judgements fall into the following areas: assessment, diagnosis and management.

Assessment

Assessment is a cognitive process which has the purpose of providing the nurse with an accurate picture of a patient's current condition (Crow, Chase & Lamond 1995). It involves the selection, collection and organization of pertinent clinical information, which the nurse then uses to make diagnostic and managerial judgements. Assessment is a dynamic process because the nurse is constantly collecting information about the patient, which may in turn lead to changes in diagnostic and managerial judgements. This is particularly so when patients are acutely ill because their condition can change so rapidly.

Interestingly, Tanner (1987) does not allude to the nursing judgements that are made during evaluation and reassessment (i.e. to what degree the patient has responded to nursing interventions and what further information needs to be collected). Indeed, evaluation and reassessment judgements tend to be overlooked by many writers. It could be argued that evaluation and reassessment involve the same activities as assessment because they have the same overall purpose (i.e. to determine the patient's current condition). Therefore, for the purpose of this chapter, the terms reassessment and evaluation are subsumed under the term assessment.

Diagnostic judgements

Diagnostic judgements are made on the basis of the information collected during assessment. Nurses normally make a number of diagnostic judgements about an individual patient (e.g. the patient has pain, the patient is emotionally distressed). This is in contrast to the single diagnostic judgements that are normally made by

---

■ BOX 4.4   Examples from the classification system of the North
             American Nursing Diagnosis Association

Pain, chronic
Oral mucous membrane, altered
Constipation
Decisional conflict
Ineffective individual coping
Divertional activity deficit

---

doctors (e.g. the patient has breast cancer). Nursing diagnostic judgements are often referred to as nursing diagnoses.

Nursing diagnosis

A nursing diagnosis has been defined as 'a clinical judgement about individual, family, or community responses to actual or potential health problems/life processes. Nursing diagnoses provide the basis for selection of nursing interventions to achieve outcomes for which the nurse is accountable' (North American Nursing Diagnosis Association 1990, p. 5). Nursing diagnosis originated in the United States in the early 1970s with the purpose of guiding and improving patient care and providing a common language to communicate the nursing process (Weber 1991). However, as with the nursing process, much confusion exists about its applicability to everyday nursing practice, particularly in countries other than the United States.

According to Gordon (1987) the term nursing diagnosis refers both to the cognitive process of diagnosing and to the diagnostic judgements reached, which are then expressed as a category label (Box 4.4). These diagnostic categories describe and classify phenomena that are of concern to nurses (Briody et al 1992). Interestingly, most of the discussion on nursing diagnosis has focused on these labels as opposed to the cognitive processes. This is demonstrated by the fact that over the past 10 years a number of other groups have developed diagnostic, interventional and outcome classification systems, the most notable of which is the International Council of Nurses' International Classification for Nursing Practice (Clarke 1996).

Many would assert that diagnostic classification systems facilitate documentation, most particularly computerized documentation. However, in order to achieve this end, a classification system should have valid categorization of data, extensive categories, a built-in review process and links with other systems. None of the currently available systems can claim to fulfil these criteria. Nevertheless, if the problems with these systems can be addressed, they offer an important means of overcoming some of the many inhibitors of documentation in nursing (Howse & Bailey 1992, Tapp 1990).

Nursing diagnoses are said to enhance the professional status and power of nurses since they focus on nurses' unique contribution to healthcare and provide evidence of nurses' diagnostic role (Roberts 1990). This is important because it is often difficult to cost the nursing component of care delivery and, therefore, to have the contribution of nursing recognized by purchasers of healthcare. However, it could be argued that developing an independent classification system, which uses a language completely different to that used by other health professionals, is not in the best interest of nursing (Lützen & Tishelman 1996). Ironically, this approach may serve to reduce nurses' professional status and power within the multidisciplinary team. This is an important consideration given the limitations of the available classification systems.

Managerial judgements

Once a diagnostic judgement has been made, the next step is to decide what are the most appropriate interventions for the patient. Such judgements are referred to as managerial judgements. According to Pellegrino (1979), the clinician needs to answer two questions in order to arrive at a correct managerial judgement for a particular patient: (1) What can be done? and (2) What should be done? There is often a difference between what is deemed scientifically to be the correct intervention (what can be done?) and what should be done for a particular patient, given the patient's particular situation at the current time (what should be done?). This is because there may be a discrepancy between what the clinician and patient believe to be the right action. For example, it may be scientifically correct for a patient with cancer to be referred to a psychologist for counselling; however, the patient may not want this because of a negative previous experience with a psychologist. A compromise needs to be found between the competing possibilities. This highlights the fact that the clinical decision-making process is often complex and uncertain in nature.

Types of managerial judgements

Kim (1983) has proposed a typology of managerial judgements in nursing. She maintains that nurses make three types of management judgements: programme, operational control and agenda (Box 4.5). Programme judgements are those that involve making a plan of action that will include goal priorities and programme content. Such judgements closely approximate the types of managerial judgements that nurses are encouraged to make when using the nursing process. Operational

---

■ BOX 4.5 **Programme, operational control and agenda management judgements**

Examples of programme judgements

When a nurse:

- Develops a teaching strategy
- Plans a patient's discharge
- Decides to monitor a patient for a particular period of time
- Develops a plan of how to care for a wound.

Examples of operational control judgements

When a nurse makes a judgement:

- To withhold, administer or change the route of a drug
- To remove an intravenous or subcutaneous cannula
- To respond to a cue during an interaction with a distressed patient
- To select a particular instrument whilst undertaking a procedure
- That no intervention is necessary.

Examples of agenda judgements

When a nurse decides:

- When to carry out specific nursing procedures during a particular shift, taking into account other activities the patient may be undertaking such as physiotherapy or going for an X-ray.
- The sequence in which nursing activities will be carried out (prioritization).

control judgements are those that identify how an action should be performed. These judgements are situationally controlled and often require immediate choices. Nurses may make a number of these judgements, with one judgement triggering off another. Thus, operational control judgements are often said to be made 'on the run'. Finally, agenda judgements are those that involve prioritizing or sequencing activities within a certain timeframe.

Kim (1983) suggests that the level of patient participation will vary according to the nature of the judgement. For example, operational control judgements require immediate attention, and do not allow much time for lengthy discussion between the nurse and patient. In addition, the gap between professional and patient knowledge may be so great for a particular judgement that only a low level of collaboration can occur. Two studies have shown that the management judgement made by nurses in their everyday clinical practice can be classified according to Kim's typology, with the majority of judgements being operational control in nature (Joseph, Matrone & Osborne 1988, Redmond 1993). However, both these studies were conducted in acute care settings and it is possible that programme judgements may predominate in other, less acute, settings. Kim's contribution to our understanding of the scope of decision-making in nursing is important because it highlights that nurses make a variety of different managerial judgements, many of which cannot be anticipated or planned for.

THEORETICAL APPROACHES TO THE STUDY OF CLINICAL DECISION-MAKING

There are two distinct theoretical approaches to the study of decision-making in nursing: the rational or cognitive approach and the interpretative phenomenological approach. It is beyond the scope of this chapter to provide an indepth analysis of these approaches, but what follows is a brief summary of each approach.

Rational approach

The rational approach, which has dominated the study of decision-making *per se*, has the purpose of either describing or prescribing how people make judgements (Carroll & Johnson 1990, Elstein & Bordage 1988). Descriptive models describe how people normally think, whereas prescriptive or normative models prescribe how we ought to think and essentially define the ideal way in which the decision-maker can achieve the most highly valued outcome. According to Baron (1988) there is a difference between the prescriptive and normative model of decision-making in that prescriptive models can help to bring the decision-maker's normal thinking processes (descriptive) into closer conformity with the ideal (normative). Most descriptive models are based on observation and, since we cannot observe thinking directly, indirect methods, such as asking people to think aloud, are employed to trace the process of thinking. Prescriptive models are based on formal mathematical or statistical techniques, such as Bayes' Theorem, which determine the optimal decision-making strategy. Statistical techniques can also be used descriptively to describe how human decisions compare with those derived from a model (Tanner 1983).

Descriptive models

Most of the research that has attempted to describe clinical decision-making from a rational perspective is based on information processing theory. This theory seeks to describe the actual processes people use when solving problems and is based on the principle of bounded or limited rationality (Newell & Simon 1972). Essentially, this principle is based on the premise that it is extremely difficult to make decisions in an entirely rational way. This is because it is rarely possible for the decision-maker to obtain complete information owing to the fact that the short-term memory has a small capacity and often there is not enough time to collect all the information required to make rational decisions.

The short-term memory is where information is received from both the external world (via the senses) and the internal mental world (long-term memory), processed and then interpreted. Since short-term memory can hold only five to nine pieces of information at any one time, it creates a bottleneck when we attempt to collect information or recall relevant information from long-term memory (Carroll & Johnson 1990). Moreover, short-term memory can hold on to information for only approximately 15–20 seconds unless some effort is made to retain it by repetition or rehearsal (Carnevali & Durand Thomas 1993). As a result, information is easily lost when further information comes in or when we are distracted. In contrast, long-term memory can store huge amounts of information about life experiences and theoretical knowledge indefinitely. However, this information is difficult to access or retrieve without the right cue or code. To overcome these constraints and preserve some degree of rationality, the decision-maker has to represent the problem in a simple way and then behave as rationally as possible within the boundary of this new representation (i.e. bounded rationality). Clearly, the potential for error is huge and the most effective problem-solver will be the one who adapts their limited information processing capacity to the complex demands of the task.

Elstein, Shulman & Sprafka (1978) used the information processing approach when undertaking an extensive series of studies on the psychology of clinical reasoning. They found that doctors commonly engaged in a strategy of hypothetico-deductive reasoning. The four major components of this reasoning process are cue acquisition, hypothesis generation, cue interpretation and hypothesis evaluation. Early hypothesis generation is central to this process and allows for clustering or chunking of cues in order to overcome the limitation of the short-term memory and to serve as a guide for subsequent data collection. This means that the search for data is simplified because only certain hypotheses will be followed up. The information processing approach has gained much acceptance in nursing and, therefore, has guided a number of studies on how nurses make decisions, which have found that the diagnostic reasoning processes of nurses could be described by the hypotheticodeductive model (Tanner et al 1987, Westfall et al 1986). However, this approach is not without its limitations. Jones (1988) maintains that, at times, it involves marked cognitive effort which makes it a poor model for clinical practice. Furthermore, in a study comparing the cognitive processes used by nurses and doctors in the postoperative administration of PRN analgesia to patients with cancer, Di Giulio & Crow (1997) found that the cognitive processes used did not conform to the pattern proposed by the information processing approach.

Normative–prescriptive models

Normative–prescriptive theories of decision-making propose that the decision-maker should make a rational choice between a number of mutually exclusive alternatives, the selection of which is based upon the probabilities and values associated with each possible outcome. According to Carroll & Johnson (1990) these theories assume that decision-makers 'have consistent preferences, know their preferences, know the alternatives available, have access to information about the consequences of selecting each alternative, and combine the information according to the expected utility rule, which discounts or weighs outcomes by their probability of occurrence' (Carroll & Johnson 1990, p. 25). It is doubtful whether these criteria are rarely, if ever, met in clinical reality.

Decision analysis One prescriptive approach used commonly to study clinical decision-making is decision analysis. This is thought to provide an objective means of examining decision-making in the light of benefits and costs to the individual and society, and is proposed as a way of assisting the clinician to make decisions under conditions of uncertainty. Decision analysis consists of a number of steps:

1. Construct a mathematical model of the decision problem. This is normally done by developing a decision tree or decision flow diagram which is made up of all the decision options (choice nodes) and their consequences (chance nodes).
2. Assign probabilities to each of the chance events (based on empirical data or clinical experience).
3. Assign values (utilities) to each potential outcome (Doubilet & McNeil 1988).

The expected utility of each strategy is then computed and the alternative with the highest overall expected value is the alternative of choice. A fourth step should follow which examines the sensitivity of this choice.

Critics of this process would contend that nursing is not amenable to decision analysis because data required for probability estimates related to nursing outcomes are unknown, and in many cases impossible to identify (Jones 1988). Moreover, it can be difficult to identify mutually exclusive decision alternatives. However, Panniers & Kellogg Walker (1994) have shown how the Delphi method can be used by nurses to preselect decision alternatives which can be subjected to decision analysis. Furthermore, Doubilet & McNeil (1988) contend that decision analysis is most applicable to those clinical questions where the results of a clinical trial are not available and that sensitivity analysis of the choice actually allows the decision-maker to deal more effectively with uncertain data. Proponents of decision analysis claim that it is useful because it clarifies the stages of the decision-making process, making any underlying assumptions and data on which the choice is based, explicit (Baumann & Deber 1989). Moreover, the decision-maker may learn a lot about their own approach to decision-making as a result of the analytical process and checking intuitions against formal rules.

Interpretative phenomenological approach

The rational approach has been criticized for ignoring the role of context, the nature of the situation, and the influence of affective factors and culture on decision-making. Such criticism has led a number of nurses, most notably Benner (1984), to study decision-making from an interpretative phenomenological perspective. According to Tanner (1993), interpretative phenomenology is used to study what nurses actually do when they undertake their everyday clinical practice and to provide a practical understanding of these activities by interpreting them, although she points out that some aspects can never be made completely explicit. Benner (1984) employed interpretative phenomenology when she applied the Dreyfus & Dreyfus (1986) model of skill acquisition to the study of nursing expertise. She found that, as expertise develops, nurses move from reliance on rule-based analytical thinking to intuitive decision-making. As a result of the work of Benner and others, intuitive thinking has emerged as a legitimate form of reasoning. Tanner (1993) has defined intuitive thinking as 'judgement without a rationale'. This does not mean that intuitive thinking is irrational. It simply means that a conscious, calculative process is not used.

According to Dreyfus & Dreyfus (1986), pattern recognition, similarity recognition, commonsense understanding, skilled know-how, sense of salience and deliberative rationality are six characteristics of intuitive thinking. Furthermore, knowing the patient, a combination of practical and theoretical knowledge, and close involvement in the situation are thought to enable the expert nurse to gain an intuitive grasp of the situation and respond appropriately to it (Benner, Tanner & Chesla 1996, Tanner 1993).

It is important to note that intuitive thinking has yet to be explicated fully and much confusion still surrounds the meaning of the term (Easen & Wilcockson 1996, King & Appleton 1997). Therein lies a problem for proponents of intuitive thinking: it may be impossible to explicate fully the meaning of intuitive thinking because it is essentially an arational process which is beyond measurement and explanation by more traditional forms of science. Hence, intuitive thinking is frequently devalued and has been derided as being irrational guesswork or, worse still, supernatural mysticism (see English 1993). It could be argued, however, that some of the characteristics of intuitive thinking can be explained by rational theories. For example, various nurses have explored the differences between expert and novice practitioners using rational approaches and have found that experts use different strategies to those of novices (Corcoran 1986, Holden & Klingner 1988, Tanner et al 1987).

According to Lamond et al (1996) these differences may be linked to the content of experts' thoughts as opposed to the cognitive processes they employ when making clinical decisions. Experts are thought to have a more organized and effectively structured knowledge base which has developed from experience. As previously mentioned, information based on theoretical knowledge and life experiences is stored in the long-term memory and is difficult to access without the right cue. Effective decision-making is dependent on retrieval of this information from the long-term memory. Gale & Marsden (1983) suggest that clinicians use a pattern-matching approach to arrive at diagnostic decisions. This approach involves the clinician recognizing forceful features, which in turn act as keys to relevant long-term memory stores. Such an approach could be considered comparable to the pattern and similarity recognition components of intuitive thinking proposed by Dreyfus & Dreyfus (1986).

Hamm (1988) has made an interesting contribution to our understanding of expert thinking. He compared Hammond's cognitive continuum theory, a general framework in which different types of thinking are related to different characteristics of tasks, with Dreyfus & Dreyfus's theory of expert thinking. According to Hammond's theory, intuitive and analytical thinking are placed at either end of a continuum. The more time available and well structured the task, the more likely it is that clinicians will use analytical thinking. In contrast, Dreyfus & Dreyfus link different types of thinking with different levels of expertise. The novice depends on analytical thinking, whereas the expert makes decisions intuitively. Both of these theories refer to the concept of analysis and intuition, but each focuses on different aspects of the context of the decision (i.e. the nature of the task or the level of expertise). As a result of his analysis, Hamm (1988) concluded that the clinician needs to recognize that there are different types of thinking which are likely to occur in some contexts but not in others, and that the context will determine which type of thinking is optimal. Thus, in some contexts the expert clinician will use analytical thinking. Tanner (1993) concurs with this viewpoint and states that, at times, analytical thinking is required, particularly when experts feel that they have not sufficiently grasped the meaning of the situation.

Despite the amount of work that has been done to elucidate the nature of expert clinical decision-making, there is still a lack of clarity surrounding the subject. Much definitional confusion exists about the term expert. For example, it is not clear whether a staff nurse who has worked for 10 years in a medical oncology setting can be called an expert or whether this term applies exclusively to advanced practitioners of cancer nursing, regardless of how much experience they have. This lack of clarity is not helped by the fact that little international consensus exists about the nature of specialist and advanced practice in nursing (International Council of Nurses 1992). However, as Benner and others have shown, a critical factor in expert (intuitive) decision-making is the possession of practical and theoretical knowledge of the situation. Thus, the ability to make intuitive judgements is dependent on the nurse having extensive clinical experience and theoretical instruction in a specialty area. This means that cancer nurses who fulfil this criteria could be called experts, regardless of what role they undertake (i.e. staff nurse or advanced practitioner).

Summary

This appraisal of rational and interpretative approaches to the study of decision-making has shown that no one theory has been investigated sufficiently to conclude that it is 'the' theory of decision-making in nursing, and all are limited in their capacity to provide a comprehensive view of the decision-making process. Nevertheless, it seems clear that we employ a range of different reasoning strategies to arrive at clinical judgements and the use of each strategy may depend on the level of expertise of the decision-maker and the nature of the decision-making task. It could be argued that a more eclectic approach to the study of decision-making is required which would acknowledge the unique contribution of different theoretical perspectives to developing a more robust understanding of clinical decision-making in nursing.

THE NURSING PROCESS

In the light of the discussion on theoretical approaches to the study of clinical decision-making, it seems appropriate to explore the theoretical underpinnings of the nursing process. A search of the nursing literature from the past 20 years will reveal a plethora of articles on the nursing process; however, as Woolley (1990) points out, the literature has 'spawned an ambiguity of terms to define this approach' (p. 110). To some it is a philosophy that emphasizes individualized, patient-centred care; to others it is merely a means of organizing care or a method of documentation (i.e. care plans). Such definitional ambiguity has led to confusion about the true purpose and nature of the nursing process (Varcoe 1996).

The nursing process was first proposed in the 1960s as a means of solving patient problems which involves four stages: assessment, planning, intervention and evaluation. At the end of this cognitive process, a written care plan is developed and modified as necessary. Unfortunately, many nurses view this written care plan as the nursing process and forget that a cognitive process must come beforehand.

The development of the nursing process was spearheaded by American nurse educators, who used the written nursing care plan as a teaching method (de la Cuesta 1983). Moreover, the nursing process emerged at a time when nurses were striving to develop their role beyond traditional parameters which emphasized the authority of doctors in decision-making and a task-centred approach to care. The process was seen as a way of establishing nurses' right to diagnose and prescribe, thus usurping doctors' sole rights to these activities and ensuring occupational control and professional advancement for nurses (Porter 1995). To bring about this advancement, nurses had to be seen to act in a rational, scientific manner, which is epitomized in the stages of the nursing process. In tangent with nurses' desire

■ BOX 4.6   Purported benefits of the nursing process

- Provides a means of identifying actual and potential health problems
- Defines specific nursing responsibilities
- Provides a unity of language
- Fosters independent nursing practice
- Demonstrates the worth of nurses
- Facilitates the development of relevant nursing theory
- Bridges the distances between different nursing ideologies
- Promotes consumer satisfaction with nursing care
- Provides a means of assessing nurses' economic contribution to care

for professional advancement was their wish to move away from institutional routines towards more individualized nursing care, which emphasized the psychosocial needs of the patient and family as well as their physical problems (Henderson 1982). The nursing process was seen as a way of achieving this end. Thus, the nursing process can be viewed as a philosophy of care, a cognitive process, a written plan of care and a means by which nurses can achieve professional advancement.

According to Suhayda & Kim (1984) the nursing process has been accepted as the foundation for nursing practice because of the way in which it structures clinical judgements within the context of nursing theory and the scientific method. A large number of other benefits have been ascribed to the nursing process (Box 4.6) (Aggleton & Chalmers 1986, Mauksch & David 1972, Miller 1985, Suhayda & Kim 1984, Yura & Walsh 1973). Interestingly, many of these benefits have also been proposed for nursing diagnosis. However, there is little, if any, evidence available to demonstrate these benefits, and it could be argued that many of the claims are mere rhetoric which have been put forward with a view to persuading nurses and others that the nursing process is a legitimate and fundamental component of nursing practice.

Critics of the nursing process point out that its linear, reductionist sequence may not incorporate all the cognitive processes that nurses actually use when they make clinical judgements (Henderson 1982, Jones & Brown 1991, Roberts, While & Fitzpatrick 1995, Tanner 1987), a criticism that is supported by the previous discussion on theoretical aspects of decision-making. In addition, if one accepts that the majority of management judgements nurses make in clinical practice are operational control in nature, then one has to ask whether it is possible to develop a plan of action to cover all of the clinical situations that nurses will meet in practice. This calls into question whether the nursing process is an adequate description of how nurses solve problems in their everyday clinical practice. Indeed, there is confusion about whether the nursing process is a description of how nurses solve problems, or a prescription for how they should (Baumann & Deber 1989). Furthermore, the written care plan is generally viewed as being overly bureaucratic, time consuming, superfluous to decision-making and, many would say, bearing little resemblance to the actual care that is given (de la Cuesta 1983, Porter 1995, Suhayda & Kim 1984). Its effectiveness as a teaching method has also been questioned (Fonteyn & Flaig Cooper 1994, Tanner 1986).

However, it is important not 'to throw out the baby with the bath water'. The nursing process has certainly made a contribution to the development of nursing theory and practice. It has highlighted the fact that nurses do make clinical judgements and solve problems in their everyday clinical practice; however, the description of this cognitive process is clearly problematic and requires development to reflect the complexity of the decision-making process. The nursing process has certainly focused attention on the need for more individualized, patient-centred approaches to care, and has helped to eradicate the assembly-line methods that were such a prevalent means of organizing nursing care in years gone by. The written care plan appears to be the most problematic aspect of the nursing process and, therefore, there is a need to consider the purpose and format of these care plans and to seek better ways of keeping a record of care and demonstrating accountability.

Overall, it seems clear that we need to reconceptualize and widen our interpretation of the nursing process (Varcoe 1996). A useful first step would be to define clearly the purposes and nature of the nursing process. Only then can we make a move beyond the dualistic and adversarial thinking that has characterized discussions about the process to date. This will enable us to retain and develop those aspects that are useful and to discard those that are not.

PRACTICAL ASPECTS OF CLINICAL DECISION-MAKING IN NURSING

The uncertain nature of the decision-making process

When making a judgement, the decision-maker seeks information about the attributes or properties of the alternatives under consideration (Carroll & Johnson 1990). When alternatives have known outcomes, the judgement is said to be made under conditions of certainty (riskless choice). On the other hand, when the outcome of the alternatives are unknown or difficult to predict, the judgement is made under conditions of uncertainty (risky choice). There is an association between the complexity of the judgement situation and the degree of uncertainty, in that the more complex the judgement, the greater the uncertainty. According to Pellegrino (1979) uncertainties exist at each step of the clinical decision-making process, some controllable, some not. This is because a number of factors contribute to these uncertainties (Box 4.7). The nature of the decision-making task, the circumstances and setting in which the judgement is made, personal attributes and abilities of the decision-maker, and the limitations inherent in human cognition are also thought to contribute to the uncertainty of the decision-making process (Luker et al 1998, Tanner 1983). We attempt to cope with this uncertainty by using different reasoning strategies; however, regardless of which of these strategies we employ, our conclusions are still open to question and can never be 100% certain.

■ BOX 4.7   **Factors contributing to the uncertainty associated with clinical decision-making**

- Methods of collecting clinical data vary widely in terms of sensitivity, specificity, reliability and accuracy, which means that a significant amount of clinical data is probabilistic in nature.
- All of the defining characteristics of a diagnostic category are not always present.
- There may be a number of alternative diagnoses possible (differential diagnoses).
- Data on effectiveness and adverse effects of interventions are not always available.
- What is scientifically deduced to be the correct intervention may not be the best one for a given patient.

Clinical information

Clinical information, or cues, are the raw data from which diagnostic and managerial judgements are made. A cue is valid when it represents the properties of what is being judged, and reliable when it is a dependable indicator of that property. Clearly, if you collect highly valid and reliable cues, you will reduce the complexity of the decision-making process.

Types of clinical information

We collect either state or contextual (situational) cues, and these in turn can be further classified as being current or historical (Box 4.8). Current cues relate to the here and now, whereas historical cues relate to any time in the past. State cues provide information about characteristics or behaviours, whereas contextual cues are situations or unchanging attributes of a person. Each type of cue plays a different role in the decision-making process. Contextual cues, particularly those that are historical, play an important role in helping the nurse to predict which problems the patient is most likely to experience (Gordon 1987). Prediction is necessary in order to narrow the 'universe of possibilities', since it is impossible to collect information about every possibility because of the constraints of time and the limitation of our short-term memory. State cues can be matched to defining characteristics of possible diagnoses, which will help the nurse arrive at a correct diagnostic decision. A number of studies have shown that current state cues are the most common cue elicited when nurses make decisions (e.g. Itano 1989, Redmond 1993).

Nurses can draw on other types of information when making decisions such as their knowledge about side-effects of treatments, what interventions worked in the past in similar situations, and the nursing policies that guide practice in a particular clinical area. They also have knowledge about how the organization works and

---

■ BOX 4.8   Examples of state and current cues

State cues

Vital signs
Perception of body image
Level of anxiety, pain or fatigue
Condition of wound
Degree of alopecia
Condition of intravenous site
Ability to expectorate sputum
Attitude towards disease
Ability to mobilize
Level of consciousness

Contextual cues

Age, sex and marital status
Length of time since surgery
Treatment regimen
Pharmacological and non-pharmacological interventions
Type and amount of information the patient has been given
Previous experience of relative dying from cancer
Degree of social support
What equipment the patient uses (e.g. ostomy product, hearing aid, zimmer frame)

the constraints that this can place on practice (e.g. knowing that the night nurse will not have time to check a chart until 1 am, that certain resources are not available, or that ward round takes place at a certain time). Thus, a large number of cues are available for use by nurses when they make clinical decisions and cues can relate to patients, their family and the clinical environment (Lamond et al 1996). It is important to remember that cues are essentially probabilistic in nature and, therefore, no cue is totally reliable. Thus, nurses should not depend on one single cue or cue type to make a decision, or errors will be made. For example, placing too much emphasis on historical contextual cues may create expectations that can bias a nurse towards a particular diagnosis.

Sources of clinical information

When making clinical judgements, nurses use information from a variety of different sources including the patient, the family, other health professionals, written notes (nursing and medical records), their own long-term memory store (knowledge of the patient, from previous experience and education), equipment (e.g. thermometer, cardiac monitor) and textbooks, articles and procedure manuals. This information can be collected by means of verbal exchange, observation, touch, smell, measurement, reading and accessing the long-term memory stores. Verbal exchange has been shown to be the most frequently used means of collecting information (Lamond et al 1996, Redmond 1993). Clearly, the patient is the most important source of verbal information.

Observation is also an important means of obtaining information about patients and their families. This data collection strategy is often used in combination with touch and smell and is of particular importance for collecting information from preverbal children and others who cannot communicate because of language difficulties or cognitive impairment. Observation is used primarily to collect information about physical characteristics (e.g. condition of skin, degree of alopecia), level of consciousness, behaviours (e.g. aggression, crying) and activities (e.g. relaxing, sleeping, mobilizing, caring for a stoma).

Measurement instruments can be used to provide objective information about signs and symptoms. We measure some signs and symptoms commonly in practice (e.g. temperature, pulse, respiration, blood pressure, urinary pH); however, instruments to measure distressing symptoms are used less commonly. Measurement instruments also provide an important means of determining the effectiveness of a particular intervention and maintaining continuity of care.

Written records do not appear to be an important source of information (Lamond et al 1996, Redmond 1993). This may reflect the fact that information is often recorded inaccurately, incompletely and inconsistently, and does not reflect the care that the patient has received. Furthermore, as nurses get to know their patients, they build up an information store about them in their long-term memory and are more likely to access their memory when they need information, as opposed to written records.

Errors of decision-making

Given the fact that clinical decision-making is an uncertain process, it is not surprising that nurses are vulnerable to making poor or incorrect judgements for which, ultimately, they are accountable. Errors of decision-making occur because of inaccurate or incomplete collection of information, poor interpretation of information, breakdowns in continuity of care, or because a nurse has used a heuristic.

■ **BOX 4.9** **Reasons for inaccurate or incomplete collection of information**

- The nurse has poor communication skills.
- Lack of time.
- Patients are sometimes reluctant to discuss their condition or may be unable to find the words that describe it adequately.
- Patients may not provide clinically relevant information because they cannot know what information is relevant to a health professional.
- Patients may be unable to express themselves as a result of cognitive impairment, excessive body weakness, or a speaking impediment.
- Patients may be unable to speak the language spoken by their carers.

Sources: Francke & Theeuwen (1994), Harrison et al (1996), Hawthorn & Redmond (1998), Heaven & Maguire (1996), Wilkie et al (1995), Wilkinson (1991)

Inaccurate or incomplete collection of information

Inaccurate or incomplete acquisition of data can lead to errors of decision-making. The reasons nurses experience problems in collecting clinical information are outlined in Box 4.9. One way of overcoming the problem of inadequate collection of data is the use of objective measurement instruments. Measurement instruments provide patients with an important means of quantifying a distressing subjective experience such as pain, anxiety or nausea. However, there is abundant evidence that nurses do not use measurement instruments commonly in clinical practice (Carr 1997, Francke et al 1996, Meurier 1998). This may be because nurses do not know which instruments are available, how to use them or, simply, because they find them too difficult and time consuming to administer. It is important to note that even the most valid, reliable and sensitive measurement instrument may not provide accurate information because you are always dependent on whether the person understands how to use the instrument, regardless of whether it is self-completed (i.e. by the patient) or administered by another person.

Poor interpretation of data

Clinical decision-making involves the interpretation of clinical information and the formulation of clinical judgements. Nurses sometimes interpret non-verbal cues incorrectly since they expect patients to manifest certain signs or behaviours and then draw inferences on the basis of their presence or absence. For example, if we expect patients in pain to manifest certain physiological signs (e.g. increased pulse, cold perspiration), vocalizations (e.g. crying and moaning), body movements (e.g. protective movement) and facial expressions (e.g. clenched teeth, closed eyes), it is not surprising that in the absence of these signs and behaviours we assume the patient is not in pain. Yet overt behaviours and signs of autonomic stimulation are not always good indicators of pain intensity or quality (Hadjistavropoulos et al 1996). This is because the expression of pain is influenced by a multitude of factors including culture, gender, beliefs, attitudes and values, degree of adaptation to pain and emotional state (Hawthorn & Redmond 1998). Moreover, patients may be using pain control behaviours such as distraction and relaxation which are very open to misinterpretation. Thus, it is easy to misinterpret the intensity of a patient's pain if assessment is based on observation alone, and this error will be prevented only by placing greater emphasis on the patient's self-report.

Previous experience with, and knowledge of, similar situations will influence nurses' ability to interpret clinical information, as will their inability to handle

CLINICAL DECISION-MAKING **77**

large amounts of data as a result of the limitation of the human short-term memory, tiredness, anxiety, or excessive intake of alcohol or medication that causes sedation, their attitudes, values and beliefs, and their sensitivity to patients' problems and needs. There is evidence that nurses with less clinical experience infer a higher degree of physical suffering than more experienced nurses (Choinière et al 1990, Mason 1981). This may be because experienced nurses become desensitized after repeated exposure to patient suffering or because the only way the nurse can cope with constant exposure to suffering is to perceive the suffering as less severe. This is problematic since nurses who are more sensitive to their patients' pain have been shown to make more accurate decisions about pain (McCaffrey & Rolling Ferrell 1997). It is ironic that some experienced nurses will become desensitized to patient suffering, since they possess more clinical knowledge than less experienced nurses, which should, in theory, enable them to make more accurate clinical judgements. Indeed, some studies have shown that experienced nurses do make more accurate assessments (Halfens, Evers & Abu-Saad 1990, Jacavone & Dostal 1992). The discrepancies may merely reflect the fact that different methodologies and definitions of expertise were used in the studies.

Nevertheless, it is important to acknowledge that an expert can still make erroneous judgements. Dreyfus & Dreyfus (1986) assert that deliberative rationality is the mechanism by which the intuitive decision-maker is protected from wrong intuitions. This is where other possible understandings of the situation are examined to confirm that the decision-maker's grasp of the situation is the best one. However, intuitions can be inaccurate because deliberative rationality cannot provide 100% protection from both the uncertainty inherent in clinical decision-making and the cognitive biases that influence this process.

The attitudes, values and beliefs held by nurses may result in nurses making generalizations and stereotyping patients or, worse still, assuming that patients share their values and beliefs. This was graphically demonstrated by Brockopp et al (1998), who found that some doctors and nurses held the belief that suffering is an essential part of being human and, therefore, pain should not be treated aggressively.

Breakdown in continuity of care

To make optimal clinical judgements, nurses need to know their patients (Prescott, Soeken & Ryan 1989). The system of organizing nursing work can facilitate nurses in getting to know their patients. For example, if a nurse is allocated to care for a patient for the duration of that patient's hospital stay, the nurse will be able to build up a relationship with the patient and will learn to recognize subtle differences in the patient's condition. However, given the fact that nurses are now working much shorter shifts, and increases in both the use of part-time staff and holiday leave entitlements, such a system can be difficult to organize and breakdowns in continuity of care may occur. Continuity of care is much easier to achieve in a community setting; however, fragmentation of care can happen as a result of poor communication between health professionals working in different healthcare settings.

Use of heuristics

There is often a discrepancy between the actual judgements made by nurses and that which has been prescribed statistically. This is because nurses use a range of heuristics when making clinical judgements which lead to them having too much confidence in their judgements and being unwilling to change their mind, even in the face of disconfirming evidence. This ultimately results in errors of both diagnostic and managerial judgement.

■ **BOX 4.10   Examples of heuristics cancer nurses might use**

- When in doubt always call a doctor.
- Always consider the patient's point of view.
- Pain is what the patient says hurts.
- All patients with cancer are anxious and are therefore in need of psychological support.

Kahneman & Tversky (1979) have studied how we infer probability and found that we make a number of consistent errors or biases in this process. As a result of their studies they have proposed that prospect theory explains how and why human choice often deviates from a normative model when making decisions under conditions of uncertainty. According to this theory, we distort probabilities and use an imagined reference point to decide whether a particular outcome is a gain or a loss. This reference point is easily influenced by irrelevant factors leading to inconsistent decision-making. This can be explained in terms of the heuristics (cognitive shortcuts or rules of thumb) we use when making judgements. Heuristics are generally easy to use compared with the sophisticated rules prescribed by normative–prescriptive theories. They facilitate decision-making because they reduce the complexity of the decision-making task by helping us to make decisions within the constraints of our limited cognitive abilities; however, they are not foolproof and can lead us to make poor decisions (see examples in Box 4.10).

Some of the general heuristics used by decision-makers which may lead to inconsistent decision-making include the representativeness heuristic, the anchoring and adjustment heuristic, and the availability heuristic. The representativeness heuristic leads us to evaluate the probability of an uncertain event by the degree to which it is similar or reflects the salient features of a case (Baron 1988). For example, if a patient presents with a number of signs and symptoms of two alternative problems, one of which occurs more commonly than the other, there is a tendency to judge both alternatives to be equally probable, instead of identifying which problem is more likely given the prior probabilities.

The availability heuristic is where we evaluate the probability of an event by thinking of examples of events that are easy to remember or have occurred recently (Baron 1988). For example, if one of your patients recently experienced a rare side-effect of treatment, it is more likely that you would suspect this side-effect in another patient with even vaguely similar symptoms. Rare and impressive cases are much easier to remember than routine ones, and this may lead to overestimation. As Pellegrino (1979) warns: 'Hoofbeats don't mean zebras, unless zebras are in the vicinity'. In Europe, a hoofbeat is much more likely to mean that a horse is in the vicinity!

Finally, the anchoring and adjustment heuristic is where we identify what is known or probable (anchor) and then estimate an unknown by adjusting from this anchor (Baron 1988). This typically results in estimates too close to the anchor and often we do not adjust the anchor as new information is obtained (Carroll & Johnson 1990). Such underadjustment can lead to overconfidence in a decision.

According to Kahneman & Tversky (1984), one's choices ought to depend on the situation itself, not on the way it is described. This principle of invariance is frequently violated by how a choice is presented or framed. The framing of information is thought to bring about a shift in the reference point, which can in turn lead us to make different decisions. Box 4.11 provides an example of two ways of framing information at a handover report. The last sentence of frame B is a powerful

■ BOX 4.11   How nurses frame information

Mr X is a 45-year-old man with advanced colorectal cancer. He is currently taking sustained release morphine 90 mg twice a day for pain and is prescribed morphine 20 mg orally or 10 mg parenterally for breakthrough pain. He has been hospitalized for the past 2 weeks and during this time he has experienced intermittent episodes of intense pain.

Frame A

'Mr X experienced numerous instances of breakthrough pain overnight. I administered 20 mg oral morphine at midnight and at 1 am. Mr X asked when he could next have some analgesia because the pain was still present. I administered 10 mg parenteral morphine at this time and Mr X slept for 2 hours; however, he awoke in pain at 3.30 am and requested more analgesia. Following a further dose of 10 mg parenteral morphine he slept for the rest of the night and says he is pain free this morning. Could you ask the doctor to review his analgesia regimen?'

Frame B

'Mr X was very demanding last night. Despite having 90 mg sustained-release morphine at 10 pm he complained of pain at midnight. I gave him 20 mg oral morphine at this time and at 1 am he demanded a further dose of analgesia. So, I gave him 10 mg parenteral morphine; however, he demanded a further dose of analgesia at 3.30 am. I think he is becoming very fond of morphine and we need to watch him carefully.'

euphemism for 'I think the patient is becoming addicted'. The mere mention of this suspicion to colleagues can lead everyone to draw a similar conclusion, despite the fact that the probability of this patient becoming addicted is less than 1% (Porter & Jick 1980). So in this situation the prior probability of addiction has been distorted. Furthermore, pre-existing myths about addiction which are held by many health professionals would influence this judgement (Hawthorn & Redmond 1988). Clearly, decision-makers need to consider prior probabilities more carefully when making decisions and also to think more critically about how their attitudes and values might influence the decision-making process.

IMPROVING CLINICAL DECISION-MAKING

Decision aids

Decision aids provide a set of unambiguous step-by-step rules which guide the management of specific patient problems. There are a number of different types of decision aids including clinical algorithms, practice guidelines, expert systems and risk assessment tools.

Clinical algorithms and practice guidelines are types of decision aids which provide a means of standardizing nursing and medical practice across a number of common conditions and are thought to be of particular value for less experienced practitioners. For example, guidelines can be developed for the management of oral complications following chemotherapy or for different types of wounds.

Expert systems are knowledge-based, interactive computer program which interpret data and make judgements similar to those of experts (Baumann & Deber 1989, Fox 1988). These systems use a set of explicit if–then rules, arrived at by a process of extracting knowledge from experts, which specify that if a certain problem exists, then certain actions should be taken (Carroll & Johnson 1990). For example, an expert system has been developed that specifies which cytotoxic drug regimen should be prescribed for a patient given the nature of their disease and other clinical parameters (Fox 1988).

Decision aids have proved useful in the area of cancer risk assessment. For example, the Gail and Claus models can be used to predict a woman's lifetime risk of getting breast cancer (Claus, Risch & Thompson 1994, Gail et al 1989). These models can be used by clinicians to help identify women at increased risk of developing breast cancer. Such a service is particularly important for women with a family history of breast cancer because they have a tendency to overestimate their risk of developing the disease. These women may experience significant psychological benefit from receiving a realistic prediction of their risk of developing breast cancer. Other risk assessment tools used in clinical practice are the Glasgow Coma Score (Teasdale, Galbraith & Clarke 1975) and the Norton Scale (Norton 1975).

As yet, few decision aids are used commonly in clinical practice, although, as health systems around the world are experiencing pressures such as rising costs and increasing demands for achieving more with less resources, it is likely that clinicians will be obliged increasingly to use these aids, since they can help reduce costs and improve the quality and consistency of decision-making. However, decision aids are not without their critics. Some would assert that they are incomplete, inflexible and do not take sufficient account of the context of the problem. This means that clinicians are still vulnerable to making incorrect judgements when using these aids and, therefore, always need to take into consideration each patient's individual circumstances before arriving at a clinical judgement.

Education

Education has an important role to play in developing the decision-making skills of nurses. However, there is some controversy as to the best way of teaching clinical decision-making to nurses. Many agree that nursing education should prepare nurses to make clinical judgements under conditions of uncertainty. According to Baron (1988) education programmes should encourage active open-mindedness where students are taught to search more openly for possibilities and encouraged to become more aware of the biases that they can bring to the decision-making process. Students can also be taught to use general heuristics designed to avoid these biases such as 'Always consider alternative possibilities' or 'Look for evidence against your first idea before making a judgement'.

A number of approaches to teaching decision-making have been proposed including problem-based learning, reflective practice, expert clinical mentors and expert systems. The use of case studies provide students with the opportunity of considering decisions in a protected environment. Such studies should vary in nature and mimic clinical reality as closely as possible. Therefore, they should include unexpected events. It is useful if the teacher is unaware of the final outcome, as in clinical reality, since the resulting uncertainty allows real clinical thinking to emerge. Reflection on practice enables students to consider their thoughts, feelings and actions surrounding a particular clinical situation and to explore the theoretical rationale for their judgements. Either undertaking a ward round or working closely with an expert nurse can provide students with the opportunity of seeing expert judgement in practice. Expert nurses can point out qualitative differences between patients who have similar problems and can prompt students to consider how diagnostic and managerial judgements might change according to different patient scenarios.

Although expert systems are still not commonly employed in clinical practice, they are thought to be extremely useful in education. This is because computer simulations allow students to make judgements in a protected, low-risk environment, unlike the real situation where an incorrect judgement can have catastrophic consequences. Indeed, if the student makes a poor judgement using the computer simulation, it may reinforce the importance of weighing up the consequences of each choice before taking action.

PATIENT INVOLVEMENT IN DECISION-MAKING

A chapter on clinical decision-making would not be complete without a discussion on patient involvement in decision-making. It is generally acknowledged that patients have the right to participate actively in judgements about their own care. This is based on the ethical principle that human beings have the right to self-determination. However, upholding the right to self-determination means that efforts should be made to determine whether or not the patient wishes to be involved in decision-making. This is important, since there is evidence to demonstrate that not all patients with cancer want to take an active role in decision-making (Beaver et al 1996, Luker et al 1995, Rothenbacher, Lutz & Porzsolt 1997, Suominen, Leino-Kilpi & Laippala 1994).

Factors influencing patients' willingness and ability to be involved in decision-making

Patient characteristics

Some patient characteristics are thought to influence their willingness and ability to be involved in decision-making. Those who are younger, female and better educated tend to want to be involved (Cassileth et al 1980, Blanchard et al 1988, Sutherland et al 1989). On the other hand, patients who are unconscious or have other cognitive impairments cannot be involved in the decision-making process, although some patients may have anticipated this situation by making a living will. A patient may not be able to access sufficient information in order to become involved in the decision-making process. Some patients have poor eyesight or hearing, which means that they cannot read small print or that they miss important pieces of information during an interaction with a health professional. A significant number of patients have low literacy skills (Doak et al 1998); others may not speak the language of the country in which they are being treated, which means that some are unable to read written materials, and others do not understand what is being said to them, a problem that is bound to get worse as the global mobility of people increases. Even when patients have the ability to access and read information, some of the information they are given is inaccurate. This problem was identified in a small study by Harris (1997), who found that staff working in a specialized oncology unit often gave patients inconsistent and inaccurate information about the side-effects of radiotherapy.

Attitudes of health professionals

A number of healthcare professionals hold paternalistic attitudes about patients becoming involved in treatment decision-making (Østergaard Thomsen et al 1993). They fear that involving patients in decision-making may highlight for them the advanced nature of their disease, thereby inducing anxiety and despair (Redmond 1998). Patients' relatives often share these attitudes, which means that even if a patient did want to be involved in decision-making they would be effectively blocked from doing so by a powerful conspiracy between health professionals and relatives. This scenario has been demonstrated in a survey of European gastro-enterologists, which found that patients are frequently not consulted regarding their treatment, nor are they fully informed about their diagnosis and prognosis, particularly if the prognosis is poor (Østergaard Thomsen et al 1993). In contrast, the gastroenterologists were much more likely to inform a patient's relatives of the patient's diagnosis and prognosis. There was a considerable north–south geo-graphical divide in the attitudes held by doctors towards the provision of informa-tion to the patient, in that gastroenterologists in northern Europe were much more likely to inform their patients fully than those in southern Europe.

Factors influencing how patients make judgements

There is often a discrepancy between the decisions that prescriptive models of decision analysis expect patients to make and those the patient actually makes (Eraker & Politser 1988). This may be because patients often use heuristics when making judgements. Moreover, many of the judgements confronting patients are new situations for which they have rarely considered their preferences, whereas an assumption underpinning prescriptive models is that people have reasonably well-defined preferences. It seems important, therefore, that some consideration is given to the heuristics that patients are thought to employ when confronted with difficult choices and the various biases that influence their preferences in decision-making.

Attitudes towards treatment

Patients with cancer hold a spectrum of contrasting attitudes towards the risks associated with various cancer treatments. For example, when asked a series of hypothetical questions about treatment outcomes, some patients would be willing to trade-off quantity versus quality of life, whereas others would be unwilling to make such a compromise. Younger patients, those who have children, and those who are being treated with curable intent and feel well tend to be less willing to trade-off length of life for quality of life. These patients would be more willing to accept toxic treatments to prolong life, even if this means that they would have to put up with very poor quality of life and, in some cases, risk immediate death. This is in stark contrast to patients who value quality of life and are therefore unwilling to compromise their quality of life, or indeed risk immediate death, in order to make long-term gains (McNeil, Weichselbaum & Pauker 1978, Perez et al 1997, Stiggelbout et al 1995, 1996).

A patient's willingness to trade-off quality versus quantity of life may be influ-enced when the level of probability of survival from a certain treatment drops. For example, O'Connor (1989) demonstrated that patients' preferences for more effec-tive toxic treatment decreased when the chance of survival dropped below 50%. This may be because, in general, people are risk-averse: we treat losses as more serious than equivalent gains and therefore tend to take risks to avoid certain losses and avoid risks to obtain a certain gain (Baron 1988). Such attitudes can clearly lead to bias when patients make judgements about treatments. However, it is not clear whether these attitudes, which are based on hypothetical situations, would change when patients are faced with actual judgements or as their physical state deteriorates.

Framing of information

A number of studies have explored whether the framing of information has an effect on the judgements made by patients with cancer (McNeil et al 1982,

■ **BOX 4.12   Examples of framing**

Frame presented in terms of probability of living

'The treatment for your cancer will involve the intravenous administration of three drugs for a 2-day period, every 21 days, for a total of 6 months. Five years after this treatment, 55 out of 100 patients will have survived.'

Frame presented in terms of probability of dying

'The treatment for your cancer will involve the intravenous administration of three drugs for a 2 day period, every 21 days, for a total of 6 months. Five years after this treatment, 45 out of 100 patients will have died.'

O'Connor 1989). In these studies information about hypothetical treatments was presented (framed) to patients in terms of probability of living (gains achieved), probability of dying (losses entailed) (Box 4.12) or probability of both living and dying. Patients tended to regard treatments presented in terms of probability of survival as more preferable than those presented in terms of probability of dying, despite the fact that the probabilities were equivalent.

O'Connor (1989) cautions that the presentation of information about treatment outcome in terms of dying, when the probability of outcome is low, may result in some patients giving up hope. She also highlights the fact that there is considerable variation in how patients respond to the framing of information. In contrast, Llewellyn-Thomas, McGreal & Thiel (1995) found no effects from framing information when patients were asked to indicate their preferences for participation in decision-making or willingness to enter a clinical trial. This may have occurred because the judgement approximated closely to a real situation and did not involve risks at the extremes of probability which, in essence, diluted the effects of framing. It is also possible that the effects of framing can be attenuated not only by the salience of the problem and the amount of specific information provided, but also by the varying attitudes patients hold towards different types of risk and the degree of interaction the patient enters into with health professionals.

The role of heuristics

Some of the heuristics patients use in decision-making may dilute the effect of framing and influence their willingness to make a judgement. McNeil et al (1982) found that when patients were asked to choose between surgery or radiotherapy on the basis of cumulative probabilities and life expectancy data, and when these therapies were identified rather than unidentified, patients had a clear preference for surgery over radiotherapy. These authors suggest that patients may rely more on pre-existing beliefs regarding treatments than on the framing of data in statistical probabilities, and this may reflect widely held misconceptions about, and bias towards, radiotherapy. Such decision-making behaviour may be based on the general heuristics of availability and vividness (Eraker and Politser 1988). Availability, as you will recall, refers to the tendency for people to judge the likelihood of an event by the ease with which related situations can be remembered. Judgements may be influenced by both direct experience and indirect exposure through the mass media. Vividness is where emotionally stimulating information has a disproportionate effect on judgements. In other words, very low probabilities are overweighed based on dramatic events or enthusiastic, and sometimes inaccurate, publicity. This may cause people to avoid a particular treatment because they have misperceived concerns about adverse events (Box 4.13).

■ BOX 4.13   Clinical examples

Availability heuristic

A women with ovarian cancer refused to have chemotherapy because her father had suffered excessively when receiving such treatment 20 years previously and she still has very distressing memories of her father's cancer experience. Her judgement was reinforced by reading a sensational article in a local newspaper about a man, with a different cancer to her, who died while receiving his third cycle of chemotherapy.

Vividness heuristic

A man with prostate cancer refused radiotherapy because he was afraid that he would become radioactive.

Loomes & Sugden (1982) proposed a modification of prospect theory to explain why human choice often deviates from a normative model, which they called regret theory. According to this theory, people regret their judgements if they learn that the outcome would have been better if they had chosen differently. We have a tendency to overweigh anticipated feelings of regret, which can lead us to make judgements that will minimize the possibility of the worst outcome occurring. For example, people with very minor complaints frequently visit their physician in order to have a disease with a very low probability of occurrence outruled. Anticipation of regret can also cause some patients to minimize their involvement in the decision-making process (Eraker & Politser 1988). To avoid regret at having made, or even contributed, to a bad judgement, the patient will devolve decision-making to the healthcare team. Thus, the healthcare team is left with the onerous responsibility of inferring patient preference in order to arrive at a correct judgement about treatment. This is particularly difficult as a number of studies have shown that the treatment preferences of patients with cancer differ considerably from those of doctors, nurses and the general public (Bremnes, Anderson & Wist 1995, Slevin et al 1990). Indeed, health professionals are often unaware of their patients' preferences (Rothenbacher, Lutz & Porzsolt 1997) and thus may make a judgement based on what they would want as opposed to what is in the best interest of the patient.

Facilitating patient decision-making in practice

The results of studies on patient involvement in decision-making have a number of implications for clinical practice. The provision of information is a fundamental component of facilitating patient participation in decision-making. The issue of information-giving is addressed in depth in Chapter 7; however, a number of points need to be made here.

Patients should be given accurate information about the disease and its treatment, and various different media should be used to help a patient understand this information. It should be recognized that some patients have particular problems accessing and understanding information; these patients should be identified and innovative strategies employed to meet their informational needs. There is evidence that informational needs change over time and, therefore, some effort is required to ensure that patients are only given the information that they need at a particular moment in time. Health professionals also need to be aware that how they present information may influence the decision a patient makes. This is important because it is unethical for health professionals to use the effects of framing to influence a patient's judgement in the direction that they wish the patient to take. However, as we are uncertain about the effects of framing in clinical reality and of the factors that might dilute these effects, this ethical dilemma may be somewhat overstated. Nevertheless, until substantive evidence is available to the contrary, it seems prudent for health professionals to remember the potential effects of framing when presenting information to a patient.

Patients differ in the degree to which they want to be involved in the decision-making process, with some wanting to be an active participant and others wanting a more passive role which may or may not involve a degree of involvement in the decision-making process. There is evidence that certain patient characteristics, such as age, influence the degree to which patients wish to participate in decision-making. However, preferences differ markedly between patients, which means that it is dangerous to generalize and stereotype them according to a particular characteristic. In addition, some patients are too unwell at a particular moment in time to want to be involved in the decision-making process, although their preference may well change once their condition improves. This suggests that decision-making preferences are unstable, and some caution is required to ensure that patients' autonomy of choice is not compromised (Waterworth & Luker 1990). Thus, assumptions about individual patient's preference for involvement in decision-making should not be made.

Patients hold a variety of attitudes towards cancer treatments, with some wishing treatment at all costs and others willing to forego active treatment in order to preserve their quality of life. Healthcare professionals' attitudes towards treatment are often considerably different from those of their patients, so great care is required to ensure that assumptions are not made about what the patient would want based on the health professional's attitude. Otherwise, the chance of making a serious error of judgement is enormous. It is also important to remember that a patient's attitude towards treatment may change over time, and efforts should be made to ensure that the patient's wishes and preferences are met as much as possible.

Finally, patients and health professionals often hold misconceptions about cancer treatments and these may have an adverse influence on decision-making. Health professionals need to become aware not only of the validity of their attitudes, values and beliefs, but also of the degree to which they influence decision-making. All the above-mentioned approaches may prove time consuming in the short term, but they will probably ease some of the burdens and uncertainties associated with clinical decision-making and have considerable benefits for the patient.

CONCLUSION

Clinical decision-making is both a complicated and controversial subject. There is no clear agreement about the nature of clinical decision-making in nursing and much work is required to clarify this situation. This may be difficult to achieve since the nursing community appears to have accepted, often without question, unsubstantiated theoretical proposals about the nature of the decision-making process. To advance the art and science of clinical decision-making in nursing, there is a need to subject both these, and novel, theoretical proposals to rigorous and critical testing. Moreover, nurses need to look critically at practical aspects of clinical decision-making to determine ways of optimizing the decision-making process and avoiding errors of judgement. Decision-making can be improved through the enhancement of clinical experience and theoretical knowledge, but more importantly by nurses becoming more aware of the impact of their attitudes, values and beliefs on the decision-making process and of the various heuristics they employ in everyday clinical practice. Facilitating nurses to achieve this end should be one of the prime goals of nurse education at all levels. Involving patients in decision-making can alleviate some of the uncertainty associated with the process; however, this is not an easy undertaking and further studies are required to elucidate the best ways of facilitating patient involvement.

REFERENCES

Aggleton P, Chalmers H 1983 Nursing models and the nursing process. Macmillan, London.
Aggleton P, Chalmers H 1986 Nursing research, nursing theory and the nursing process. Journal of Advanced Nursing 11:197–202
Bandman E L, Bandman B 1995 Critical thinking in nursing, 2nd edn. Appleton & Lange, Norwalk, Connecticut
Baron J 1988 Thinking and deciding. Cambridge University Press, Cambridge
Baumann A, Deber R 1989 Decision making and problem solving in nursing: an overview of the relevant literature. Literature Review Monograph 3, University of Toronto, Toronto
Beaver K, Luker K A, Glynn Owens R, Leinster S J, Degner L F 1996 Treatment decision making in women newly diagnosed with breast cancer. Cancer Nursing 19(1):8–19
Benner P 1984 From novice to expert: excellence and power in clinical nursing practice. Addison-Wesley, Menlo Park, California
Benner P, Tanner C, Chesla C 1996 Expertise in nursing practice. Caring, clinical judgement and ethics. Springer, New York
Blanchard C G, Lebrecque M S, Ruckdeschel J C, Blanchard E B 1988 Information and decision-making preferences of hospitalized adult cancer patients. Social Science and Medicine 27:1139–1145
Bremnes R M, Andersen K, Wist E A 1995 Cancer patients, doctors and nurses vary in their willingness to undertake cancer chemotherapy. European Journal of Cancer 31A(12):1955–1959
Briody M E, Carpenito L J, Jones D A, Fitzpatrick J J 1992 Towards further understanding of nursing diagnosis: an interpretation. Nursing Diagnosis 3(3):124–128
Brockopp D Y, Brockopp G, Warden S, Wilson J, Carpenter J S, Vandeveer B 1998 Barriers to change: a pain management project. International Journal of Nursing Studies 35:226–232
Carnevali D L, Durand Thomas M 1993 Diagnostic reasoning and treatment decision making. J B Lippincott, Philadelphia
Carr E C J 1997 Evaluating the use of a pain assessment tool and care plan: a pilot study. Journal of Advanced Nursing 26:1073–1079
Carroll J, Johnson E 1990 Decision research: a field guide. Sage Publications, Beverly Hills, California
Cassileth B R, Zupkis R V, Sutton-Smith K, March V 1980 Information and participation preference among cancer patients. Annals of Internal Medicine 92:832–836
Chinn P, Jacobs M 1983 Theory and nursing: a systematic approach. C V Mosby, St Louis
Choinière M, Melzack R, Girard N, Rondeau J, Paquin M-J 1990 Comparisons between patients' and nurses' assessment of pain and medication efficacy in severe burn injuries. Pain 40:143–152
Clarke J 1996 How nurses can participate in the development of an ICNP. International Nursing Review 43(6):171–174
Claus E B, Risch N, Thompson D 1994 Autosomal dominant inheritance of early-onset breast cancer: implications for risk prediction. Cancer 73:645–651
Corcoran S 1986 Task complexity and nursing expertise as factors in decision making. Nursing Research 35(2):107–112
Crow R, Chase J, Lamond D 1995 The cognitive component of nursing assessment: an analysis. Journal of Advanced Nursing 22:206–212
de la Cuesta C 1983 The nursing process: from development to implementation. Journal of Advanced Nursing 8:365–371
Di Giulio P, Crow R 1997 Cognitive processes nurses and doctors use in the administration of PRN (at need) analgesic drugs. Scandinavian Journal of Caring Sciences 11:12–19
Doak C C, Doak L G, Friedell G H, Meade C D 1998 Improving comprehension for cancer patients with low literacy skills: strategies for clinicians. CA: A Cancer Journal for Clinicians 48:151–162

Doubilet P, McNeil B J 1988 Clinical decisionmaking. In: Dowie J, Elstein A (eds) Professional judgement: a reader in clinical decision making. Cambridge University Press, Cambridge, ch 13, p 255

Dreyfus H, Dreyfus S 1986 Mind over machine. Free Press, New York

Easen P, Wilcockson J 1996 Intuition and rational decision making in professional thinking: a false dichotomy? Journal of Advanced Nursing 24:667–673

Elstein A S, Bordage G 1988 Psychology of clinical reasoning. In: Dowie J, Elstein A (eds) Professional judgement: a reader in clinical decision making. Cambridge University Press, Cambridge, ch 4, p 109

Elstein A, Shulman L, Sprafka S 1978 Medical problem solving: an analysis of clinical reasoning. Harvard University Press, Cambridge

English I 1993 Intuition as a function of the expert nurse: a critique of Benner's novice to expert model. Journal of Advanced Nursing 18:387–393

Eraker S A, Politser P 1988 How decisions are reached: physician and patient. In: Dowie J, Elstein A (eds) Professional judgement: a reader in clinical decision making. Cambridge University Press, Cambridge, ch 20, p 379

Fonteyn G, Flaig Cooper L 1994 The written nursing process: is it still useful to nursing education? Journal of Advanced Nursing 19(3):315–319

Fox J 1988 Formal and knowledge-based methods in decision technology. In: Dowie J, Elstein A (eds) Professional judgement: a reader in clinical decision making. Cambridge University Press, Cambridge, ch 12, p 226

Francke A L, Theeuwen I 1994 Inhibition in expressing pain: a qualitative study among Dutch surgical breast cancer patients. Cancer Nursing 17(3):193–199

Francke A L, Garssen B, Abu-Saad H H, Grypdonck M 1996 Qualitative needs assessment prior to a continuing education programme. Journal of Continuing Education in Nursing 27(1):34–41

Gail M H, Brinton L A, Byar D P et al 1989 Projecting individualised probabilities of developing breast cancer for white females who are being examined annually. Journal of the National Cancer Institute 81:1879–1886

Gale J, Marsden P 1983 Medical diagnosis: from student to clinician. Oxford University Press, Oxford

Gordon M 1987 Nursing diagnosis: process and application. McGraw-Hill, New York

Hadjistavropoulos H D, Craig K D, Hadjistavropoulos T, Poole G D 1996 Subjective judgements of deception in pain expression: accuracy and errors. Pain 65:251–258

Halfens R, Evers G, Abu-Saad H 1990 Determinants of pain assessment by nurses. International Journal of Nursing Studies 27(1):43–49

Hamm R M 1988 Clinical intuition and clinical analysis: expertise and the clinical continuum. In: Dowie J, Elstein A (eds) Professional judgement: a reader in clinical decision making. Cambridge University Press, Cambridge, ch 3, p 78

Harris R L 1997 Consistency of patient information … is this happening? Cancer Nursing 20(4):274–276

Harrison A, Ahmed Busabir A, Obeid Al-Kaabi A, Khalid Al-Awadi H 1996 Does sharing a mother-tongue affect how closely patients and nurses agree when rating the patient's pain, worry and knowledge? Journal of Advanced Nursing 24:229–235

Hawthorn J, Redmond K 1998 Pain: causes and management. Blackwell Science, Oxford

Heaven C M, Maguire P 1996 Training hospice nurses to elicit patient concerns. Journal of Advanced Nursing 23:280–286

Henderson V 1982 The nursing process – is the title right? Journal of Advanced Nursing 7:103–109

Holden G, Klingner A 1988 Learning from experience: differences in how novices vs. expert nurses diagnose why an infant is crying. Journal of Nursing Education 27(1):23–29

Howse E, Bailey J 1992 Resistance to documentation – a nursing research issue. International Journal of Nursing Studies 29(4):371–380

International Council of Nurses 1992 Specialisation in nursing. ICN, Geneva

Itano J 1989 A comparison of the clinical judgement process in experienced registered nurses and student nurses. Journal of Nursing Education 28(3):120–126

Jacavone J, Dostal M 1992 A descriptive study of nursing judgement in the assessment and management of cardiac pain. Advances in Nursing Science 15(1):54–63

Jones J 1988 Clinical reasoning in nursing. Journal of Advanced Nursing 13:185–192

Jones S, Brown L 1991 Critical thinking: impact on nursing education. Journal of Advanced Nursing 16:529–533

Joseph D, Matrone J, Osborne E 1988 Actual decision making: factors that determine practices in clinical settings. Canadian Journal of Nursing Research 20(2):19–31

Kahneman D, Tversky A 1979 Prospect theory: an analysis of decisions under risk. Econometrica 47:263–291

Kahneman D, Tversky A 1984 Choices, values, and frames. American Psychologist 39:341–350

Kim H 1983 Collaborative decision making in nursing practice: a theoretical framework. In: Chinn P (ed) Advances in nursing theory development. Aspen Systems, Rockville, p 271

King L, Appleton J V 1997 Intuition: a critical review of the research and rhetoric. Journal of Advanced Nursing 26:194–202

Lamond D, Crow R, Chase J, Doggen K, Swinkels M 1996 Information sources used in decision making: considerations for simulation development. International Journal of Nursing Studies 33(1):47–57

Llewellyn-Thomas H A, McGreal J, Thiel E C 1995 Cancer patients' decision making and trial-entry preferences: the effects of 'framing' information about short-term toxicity and long-term survival. Medical Decision Making 15:4–12

Loomes G, Sugden R 1982 Regret theory: an alternative theory of rational choice under uncertainty. Economic Journal 92:805–824

Luker K A, Beaver K, Leinster S J, Glynn Owens R, Degner L F, Sloan J A 1995 The information needs of women newly diagnosed with breast cancer. Journal of Advanced Nursing 22:134–141

Luker K A, Hogg C, Austin L, Ferguson B, Smith K 1998 Decision making: the context of nurse prescribing. Journal of Advanced Nursing 27:657–665

Lützen K, Tishelman C 1996 Nursing diagnosis: a critical analysis of underlying assumptions. International Journal of Nursing Studies 33(2):190–200

Mason D J 1981 An investigation of the influences of selected factors on nurses' inferences of patient suffering. International Journal of Nursing Studies 18(4):251–259

Mauksch I, David M 1972 Prescription for survival. American Journal of Nursing 72(12): 2189–2193

McCaffrey M, Rolling Ferrell B 1997 Influences of professional vs. personal role on pain assessment and use of opioids. Journal of Continuing Education in Nursing 28(2):69–77

McNeil B J, Weichselbaum R, Pauker S G 1978 Fallacy of the five-year survival rate in lung cancer. New England Journal of Medicine 299:1397–1401

McNeil B J, Pauker S G, Sox H C, Tversky A 1982 On the elicitation of preferences for alternative therapies. New England Journal of Medicine 306:1259–1262

Meurier C E 1998 The quality of assessment of patients with chest pain: the development of a questionnaire to audit the nursing assessment record of patients with chest pain. Journal of Advanced Nursing 27:140–146

Miller A 1985 Does the process help the patient? Nursing Times 81:26

Newell A, Simon H 1972 Human problem solving. Prentice Hall, Englewood Cliffs, New Jersey

North American Nursing Diagnosis Association 1990 Taxonomy I revised. NANDA, St Louis, MO

Norton D 1975 Research and the problem of pressure sores. Nursing Mirror 140(7):65–67

O'Connor A M 1989 Effects of framing and level of probability on patients' preferences for cancer chemotherapy. Journal of Clinical Epidemiology 42(2):119–126

Østergaard Thomsen O, Wulff H R, Martin A, Singer P A 1993 What do gastroenterologists in Europe tell cancer patients? Lancet 341:473–476

Panniers T L, Kellogg Walker E 1994 A decision-analytic approach to clinical nursing. Nursing Research 43(4):245–249.

Pellegrino E 1979 The anatomy of clinical judgement. In: Engelhardt HT, Spicker S F, Towers B (eds) Clinical judgement: a critical appraisal. Reidal, Dordrecht, p 169

Perez D J, McGee R, Campbell A V, Christensen E A, Williams S 1997 A comparison of time trade-off and quality of life measures in patients with advanced cancer. Quality of Life Research 6:133–138

Porter J, Jick H 1980 Addiction rare in patients treated with narcotics. New England Journal of Medicine 302(2):123

Porter S 1995 Northern nursing: the limits of idealism. Irish Journal of Sociology 5:22–42

Prescott P A, Soeken K L, Ryan J W 1989 Measuring patient intensity: a reliability study. Evaluation & The Health Professions 12(3):255–269

Redmond K 1993 An exploratory study of the clinical judgements made by cancer nurses. MSc thesis, University of Surrey, Guildford

Redmond K 1998 Assessing patients' needs and preferences in the management of advanced colorectal cancer. British Journal of Cancer 77(suppl 2):5–7

Roberts J, While A, Fitzpatrick J 1995 Information-seeking strategies and data utilisation: theory and practice. International Journal of Nursing Studies 32(6):601–611

Roberts S L 1990 Achieving professional autonomy through nursing diagnosis and nursing DRGs. Nursing Administration Quarterly 14(4):54–60

Rothenbacher D, Lutz M P, Porzsolt F 1997 Treatment decisions in palliative cancer care: patients' preferences for involvement and doctors' knowledge about it. European Journal of Cancer 33:1184–1189

Slevin M L, Stubbs L, Plant H J et al 1990 Attitudes to chemotherapy: comparing views of patients with cancer with those of doctors, nurses, and general public. British Journal of Medicine 300:1458–1460

Stiggelbout A M, Kiebert G M, Kievit J, Leer J-W H, Harbema J D F, De Haes J C J M 1995 The 'utility' of the time trade-off method in cancer patients: feasibility and proportional trade-off. Journal of Clinical Epidemiology 48(10):1207–1214

Stiggelbout A M, De Haes J C J M, Kieber G M, Kievit J, Leer J-W H 1996 Tradeoffs between quality and quantity of life: development of the QQ questionnaire for cancer patient attitudes. Medical Decision Making 16:184–192

Suhayda R, Kim M 1984 Documentation of the nursing process in critical care. In: Kim M, McFarland G, McLane A (eds) Classification of nursing diagnosis: proceedings of the fifth national conference. C V Mosby, St Louis, p 166

Suominen T, Leino-Kilpi H, Laippala P 1994 Nurses' role in informing breast cancer patients: a comparison between patients' and nurses' opinions. Journal of Advanced Nursing 19:6–11

Sutherland H J, Llewellyn-Thomas H A, Lockwood G A, Tritchler D L 1989 Cancer patients and their desire for information and participation in treatment decisions. Journal of the Royal Society of Medicine 82:260–263

Tanner C 1983 Research on clinical judgement. In: Holzemer W (ed.) Review of research in nursing education. Stack, New Jersey

Tanner C 1986 The nursing care plan as a teaching method: reason or ritual? Nurse Educator 11(4):8–10

Tanner C 1987 Teaching clinical judgement. Annual Review of Nursing Research 5:153–173

Tanner C 1993 Rethinking clinical judgement. In: Diekelmann N L, Rather M L (eds) Transforming RN education: dialogue and debate. National League for Nursing, New York, p 15

Tanner C, Patrick K, Westfall U, Putzier D 1987 Diagnostic reasoning strategies of nurse and nursing students. Nursing Research 36:358–363

Tapp R A 1990 Inhibitors and facilitators to documentation of nursing practice. Western Journal of Nursing Research 12(2):229–240

Teasdale G, Galbraith S, Clarke K 1975 Acute impairment of brain function – 2: observation record chart. Nursing Times 7(25):972–973

Varcoe C 1996 Disparagement of the nursing process: the new dogma? Journal of Advanced Nursing 23:120–125

Waterworth S, Luker K A 1990 Reluctant collaborators: do patients want to be involved in decisions concerning care? Journal of Advanced Nursing 15:971–976

Weber G J 1991 Nursing diagnosis: a comparison of nursing textbook approaches. Nurse Educator 16(2):22–27

Westfall U E, Tanner C A, Putzier D J, Podrick K P 1986 Activating clinical inferences: a component of diagnostic reasoning in nursing. Research in Nursing and Health 9:269–277

Wilkie D, Williams A R, Grevstad P, Mekwa J 1995 Coaching persons with lung cancer to report sensory pain. Cancer Nursing 18(1):7–15

Wilkinson S 1991 Factors which influence how nurses communicate with cancer patients. Journal of Advanced Nursing 16:677–688

Woolley N 1990 Nursing diagnosis: exploring the factors which may influence the reasoning process. Journal of Advanced Nursing 15:110–117

Yates J F 1990 Judgement and decision making. Prentice-Hall, London

Yura H, Walsh M 1973 The nursing process: assessing, planning, implementing and evaluating, 2nd edn. Appleton-Century-Croft, New York

Nursing education in cancer care

Nora Kearney

CHAPTER 5

INTRODUCTION

Whilst education is undoubtedly the key to developing nursing, whatever the specialty, it cannot do so in isolation. For education to be effective it must be firmly rooted in practice and not driven by academic ideals. Education without experience will, of course, increase knowledge but education in tandem with experience has the potential to improve outcomes for individuals with cancer. It almost seems redundant to state that the care of patients with cancer requires nurses to be adequately and appropriately educated (Jodrell 1996, Royal College of Nursing Cancer Nursing Society 1996a). However, it appears that this is by no means universally accepted and much variation exists in both the educational preparation of cancer nurses and the education itself (Copp 1988, Jodrell 1996). This chapter considers the role of education in cancer nursing, the potential impact of education in cancer care, and possible directions for the future.

Differences in the way cancer is treated across Europe elicit different outcomes, and McVie (1996) contends that around 100 000 deaths from cancer could be prevented if there was more dissemination of information and more equitable access to technical and medical expertise across the continent. In terms of nursing practice little is known of how variations in practice affect individual patient outcomes but it is likely that, as with our medical colleagues, variations in clinical nursing expertise and knowledge have a detrimental effect on patient care. It would appear that at the core of these variations in practice is the lack of consistency in cancer nursing education.

A lack of cancer nursing education exists in Europe today despite the fact that in 1986 a report from the Commission of the European Communities concerning the state of cancer in Europe identified the area of training in oncology for nurses as a priority (Commission of the European Communities 1986). This identification of education in cancer nursing as a priority reflected a general trend towards an increased emphasis on continuing education in nursing generally. In 1988 the Advisory Committee on Training in Nursing (ACTN) in Europe developed recommendations concerning cancer training for nurses. Following this, in 1989, the Commission adopted a recommendation concerning the training of health personnel in the area of cancer which included the recommendations of the ACTN (European Commission 1989).

DELIVERY OF CANCER CARE

For the first time, the American Cancer Society's Department of Epidemiology and Surveillance has reported a favourable change in direction in relation to the statistics associated with cancer. They have recorded a reduction in the total number of new cancer cases and declining cancer death rates in the USA, and in addition state that 5-year survival rates are, with the exception of lung and bronchus, continuing to improve (Rosenthal 1998). However, despite this encouraging news, cancer remains a major health problem and will continue to pose significant challenges to both healthcare professionals and those responsible for financing healthcare.

The ever-increasing demands on healthcare and the reported reduction in available resources result in increasing pressure to provide optimal treatment in a cost-efficient way. Consideration of cancer care and the way in which scientific knowledge is developing subsequently presents us with somewhat of a dichotomy. On the one hand we need to reduce the cost of cancer care and on the other, new developments and technological advances require greater investment. As nurses caring for patients in this arena it is vital that we are aware of the value of cancer therapy not just in terms of survival but also in terms of the quality of that survival for individual patients and that we practise efficiently.

Much has been promised concerning the reduction in cancer deaths at an international level from organizations such as the American Cancer Society (Rosenthal 1998) and the European Commission (EC) (Commission of the European Communities 1986) and, although there may be encouraging news in terms of a downward trend, this decrease is much slower than many would like. As a consequence the search for innovative cancer therapies continues apace, with research ongoing in a number of areas, including new surgical and radiotherapy techniques, genetic manipulation and new cytotoxic agents which are addressing numerous targets. Such activity means that cancer nursing is undoubtedly a dynamic specialty. Education, therefore, must reflect the pace with which cancer management is progressing and ensure that cancer nurses have the skills and knowledge to provide optimal cancer care. The ability to provide the best possible nursing care is multi-faceted and educationalists are obliged to consider this diversity when undertaking curriculum development.

In addition, the provision of care for people with cancer depends not only on the healthcare professionals involved in delivering care but must also reflect trends in healthcare, the economic situation, the particular politics of the day, and the attitudes and values of society. In Europe this is by no means straightforward but, with the growing harmonization of Europe, recently exemplified by economic and monetary union, it is likely that healthcare will also benefit from closer collaboration.

CANCER NURSING EDUCATION

The development of cancer nursing education in Europe has occurred in a piece-meal fashion despite the recommendations from the EC and ACTN. This is most likely due to the fact that what was delivered by the Commission in 1989 were merely recommendations and not policy. As a consequence few member states adopted these recommendations and the development of cancer nursing education at a postbasic level has been carried out predominantly by a small number of committed individuals working independently within institutions.

Probably the most notable educational development in Europe regarding cancer nursing education was the development of the 'core curriculum for a postbasic course in cancer nursing' (European Oncology Nursing Society 1990). This was developed under the auspices of the European Oncology Nursing Society (EONS) with funding from the EC's Europe Against Cancer Programme. Following the development of the curriculum, a consensus meeting was held with individuals involved in education and practice from throughout Europe, thus ensuring the applicability of the curriculum across Europe. Since its production in 1990 the curriculum has been utilized in over 13 countries as the basis for educational development (Jodrell 1996). As with any tool to be used at a European level, the curriculum was developed to meet the needs of those just beginning to develop education in cancer nursing while offering a structure to those with developed programmes. A review of cancer nursing education which had been funded by the Europe Against Cancer Programme during 1990 and 1994 demonstrated that the majority of courses for nurses were developed across Europe using the curriculum as a framework (Jodrell 1997). However, the review also recommended that the curriculum be updated and, with support from the EC, a new curriculum has been developed.

The second edition of the curriculum (EONS 1999) is more comprehensive than the original, and is based on patient and family need. The curriculum was developed in collaboration with the Royal College of Nursing Paediatric Oncology Nursing Forum and the International Society of Paediatric Oncology (SIOP Europe) and reflects a consensus between representatives from all member states of the European Union. In addition to this, EONS, with support from the Europe Against Cancer Programme, is working in collaboration with the European Quality Assurance Nurses Group (EUROQUAN) to produce a framework for developing education at an advanced level. The result of this work will be the

Table 5.1 Courses organized in the European Union 1990–1994

Country	No. of courses	Total no. of nurses	Length of course
Belgium	6	122	30 weeks
		118	
		162	30 weeks
		Not specified	
		38	3 weeks
		80	30 weeks
Denmark	4	26	s1 week
		20	33 weeks
		61	5 days per module
		162	
Greece	6	137	1 week
		15	7 months
		110	1 week
		13	7 months
		14	7 months
		47–186	1–2 days
Germany	2	14	1 year
		18	1 year
Ireland	2	25	
		61	5 days
Luxembourg	1	5	8–12 weeks
Italy	5	51	30 weeks
		40	Not specified
		28	Not specified
		40	Not specified
		Not specified	
Portugal		Not specified	18 months
	4	28	12 months
		41	14 weeks
		40	7 weeks
Spain		100	2 weeks
	3	Not specified	Not specified
		100	Not specified

development of a framework for a curriculum for advanced cancer nursing practice and the production of outcome standards for cancer nursing practice.

The extensive review of cancer nursing education supported by the EC (Jodrell 1997) identified the level of variability in the provision of postbasic cancer nursing education in Europe. Table 5.1 highlights the inconsistency with which cancer nursing education programmes are developed.

The average duration for courses was around 7 months, but ranged from 1 week to 18 months. This level of inconsistency is difficult to interpret especially since all the programmes claimed to be based on the core curriculum for a postbasic course in cancer nursing developed by EONS. From further interviews with organizers of these courses it was evident that the duration of the course had more to do with resource allocation than educational need.

Cancer nurse education is required to meet the needs of nurses at different levels and is a feature of both basic nurse training courses and of specialized postbasic courses. Considerable variation exists in terms of the emphasis given to cancer education, time allocated to it and the way it is taught. Studies in Europe and America investigating the cancer content of nurse education programmes report similar findings and make a number of recommendations relating to proposed changes (Copp 1988, Pope 1992). These are summarized in Box 5.1.

BASIC NURSE EDUCATION

In 1991 the Standing Committee of Nurses in Europe (PCN) received funding from the European Commission to undertake a project to establish guidelines for the cancer content in basic nursing education programmes in Europe (Europe Against Cancer Programme project no. SOC 92 000227). The project involving 11 member states held an initial workshop in 1992 and made the following recommendations:

1. Guidelines should be based on the ACTN report and Recommendations on Training in Cancer (III/D/248/3/88) and pp. 2–3 of 'A core curriculum for a post basic course in cancer nursing' (EONS 1990), adjusted to national conditions.
2. Inappropriate to determine the number of hours required.
3. Local decisions required regarding the nature of integrating theory and practice.
4. Increased emphasis on prevention and community.
5. Levels of competence and scope of practice to be clarified.
6. Clarification of specialism necessary.
7. Necessary to determine the required educational outcome.

■ **BOX 5.1** **Content of cancer nursing education programmes (adapted from Pope 1992)**

Recommendations:
- Concept of cancer nursing should be contained in all education programmes.
- Curricula should be evaluated to ensure they reflect the dynamic nature of the specialty of oncology.
- There are specific areas of knowledge that must be addressed in any cancer nursing programme (basic science of cancer, specific care of patients, cancer in society, psychological support and palliative care).
- Expert cancer nurses should be involved in delivering the programme.
- The programme should include transferable skills.
- Clinical experience in an oncology area is important.
- Updating of knowledge is vital for all cancer nurses.

Following these recommendations each member state held their own national workshops to develop new educational material on the teaching of cancer at basic level, based on the guidelines agreed at the European workshop and identified above. These guidelines have been incorporated into basic education in the majority of member states (Standing Committee of Nurses of the EU 1995).

POSTBASIC EDUCATION

Before the development of the core curriculum (EONS 1990), there was no available framework for nurse educators in Europe wishing to develop cancer nursing education. Whilst not comprehensive, the curriculum did offer educationalists a basis from which to build their own programmes. It also provided cancer nurses in Europe with a tool with which to lobby at a national level for the development of education programmes in cancer nursing, which had hitherto not been available.

Over the past few years there has been a growing recognition of the need for educated nurses to deliver increasingly complex cancer care (Expert Advisory Group on Cancer 1995, Royal College of Nursing Cancer Nursing Society 1996b). Yet, in the majority of countries in Europe, there is no clear strategy for education delivery (Jodrell 1997) and frameworks for professional development are lacking. In the UK the regulatory body for nurses, the United Kingdom Central Council for nurses (UKCC), has identified that some form of education is important (UKCC 1994), but there remains confusion over educational level for advanced practice.

This disparity probably reflects the conflicting opinions that currently exist in relation to academic levels in nursing. Davis & Burnard (1992) offer some advice when considering the characteristics that differentiate different levels of academic study (Table 5.2).

Whilst such information is useful, the lack of any formalized and recognized pathway means that lack of clarity remains for nurses wishing to access education in order to advance practice. In the USA there appears to be a much clearer pathway for nurses wishing to function as clinical nurse specialists or nurse practitioners. Nurses wishing to practise at this level would be expected to have undertaken further education, usually at Master's level (American Nurses Association 1980). However, nowhere in Europe is there clear guidance, let alone policy, for nurses in such advanced roles. Given the variation in nursing practice that currently exists in Europe (Salvage 1997), it has been suggested that it would perhaps be more

Table 5.2 Characteristic differences between levels of educational preparation (adapted from Davis & Burnard 1992)

	Diploma level	Bachelor's degree	Master's degree	Doctoral degree
Characteristics of knowledge	Broad base; discrete categories	Broad and deep; integration across categories	Narrow and deep	Very specific; generation of new knowledge
Nature of research studies	Introduction	Utilization of research findings	Competence in research methods	Advanced research skills
Teacher–student relationship	Teacher–student contact high	Beginning of independent study	Partnership but with structure curriculum	Supervisory
Locus of control	With tutor	Negotiated	With tutor	With student

appropriate to focus on the attributes required to advance practice rather than the educational level required (Knowles & Kearney 1998). If this is the case at present, it remains that we must work towards establishing definitive criteria for educational preparation for cancer nurses working at an advanced level.

EDUCATION TO ADVANCE PRACTICE

The notion that education is not required to advance practice seems somewhat of an anathema, yet there remains, in many countries, little recognition of the importance of such education. This may be the result of a perceived lack of evidence that educating nurses makes a difference to patient outcomes, and nurses themselves have to address this problem through research and educational initiatives. The rationale behind education for advanced practice is often questioned in nursing and it seems that we have learnt little from early educationalists such as Yeaxlee, who stated in 1929: 'To ask whether a man should be a student for the sake of knowledge he acquires or for the sake of the qualities he develops in the course of particular studies is to raise a false dilemma. Each has its own importance but neither is separable from the other' (p. 142). It could be argued that this statement remains poignantly relevant today for nurses wishing to undertake education to advance practice.

It has been claimed that a major discrepancy between specialist nurses practising in North America compared with countries in Europe, such as the UK, is their educational preparation. The American Nurses Association Congress of Nursing Practice defines a nurse practising at an advanced level (e.g. clinical nurse specialist) as a registered nurse 'who through study and supervised practice at the graduate level (Master's or doctorate) has become expert in a defined area of knowledge and practice in a selected area of nursing' (American Nurses Association 1980). In Europe educational criteria for advanced practice have not been defined and as a consequence the educational preparation of nurses working in advanced practice roles is extremely variable, and indeed in some countries is non-existent. Given this reality, then, it is unlikely that at present we could stipulate a mandate for educational preparation for advanced practice. However, the recognition that education and training of registered nurses is associated with good quality care must surely mean that moving in this direction is a priority for cancer nurse education in Europe.

The difficulty in recognizing advanced education within specialized areas such as cancer nursing may result from the lack of clarification that surrounds advanced practitioner roles. As suggested by Hamric (1995), the nursing profession must measure the outcomes, in relation to patient benefit, of advanced practitioner roles in order that administrators not only value but also support the role. Defining, articulating and understanding advanced practitioner roles while demonstrating outcomes of advanced practice may lead to the justification of what the necessary educational preparation should be.

Anecdotal evidence would suggest that nurses themselves are seeking clarification of what constitutes advanced practice and exactly what educational preparation is required to provide optimal nursing care. However, without clear guidance and support from senior nurses involved with policy changes, it remains that the *ad hoc* development of advanced practice will continue. In addition, the little research available in this area demonstrates that whilst clinically based nurses wish to undertake education to advance practice they receive limited support from managers (Jodrell 1996) and policy-makers (Jodrell 1997). This is despite the fact that policy-makers have clearly stated that the delivery of cancer care should be carried out by nurses who have benefited from postbasic cancer nursing education (Expert Advisory Group on Cancer 1995).

PREPARATION OF CANCER NURSES

It has been identified by numerous researchers that nurses do not receive adequate preparation to deliver effective care to patients with cancer (Corner & Wilson-Barnett 1992, Jodrell 1996) and that barriers exist to the implementation of new knowledge in the clinical area (Sneddon 1992). In addition, further studies have shown that nurses who have not benefited from postbasic education in cancer nursing experience more stress related to nursing patients with advanced cancer (Wilkinson 1986). Added to this is the evidence that nurses who have completed postbasic education in cancer nursing are better facilitators of communication than those who have not undertaken such education (Wilkinson 1991).

It is vital that nurses have the opportunity to develop both educationally and clinically as a result of an educational programme. However, professional socialization studies indicate that nursing students are often confused between what they learn in schools and what is expected of them in practice (Kelly 1991). This may result in rejection of the knowledge they have gained (Sneddon 1992, Wouters 1994). The ideal must be that students themselves (at all levels) should experience real contact with a cancer care environment in which all professionals involved demonstrate appropriate levels of care and the importance of the multidisciplinary team. Such a supportive environment may produce knowledgeable practitioners with the ability to impact patient outcomes positively.

IMPACT OF NURSES IN CANCER CARE

The effectiveness of specialist nurses in cancer care has been demonstrated (James, Gurrero & Brada 1994, Maguire et al 1980, McArdle et al 1996, Palsson & Norberg 1995, Watson et al 1988). In addition, the role of cancer nurses in the clinical trial setting is undisputed (Lake & Jenkins 1993, Pfister-Minogue 1993, Rich 1993) and evidence is accumulating on the impact of nursing interventions on patient outcomes (Corner et al 1996, Faithfull 1995, Preston 1995). What is clear form the majority of these studies, and particularly from the most recent work from Corner's group, is that such effectiveness is gained by employing educated nurses. This recent work supports the growing body of literature that is emerging regarding the effectiveness of nurse-led interventions from a range of health settings, including management of acute pain (Mackintosh & Bowles 1997), urinary incontinence (O'Brian et al 1991), diabetes care (Mallows et al 1990) and stoma care (Wade 1990).

That educated nurses have an impact on care has been demonstrated (Carr-Hill et al 1992). However, to add weight to this argument, nurse educators need to consider the evaluation of educational programmes and ensure that they clearly identify the benefits to patient outcomes resulting from such programmes.

EVALUATION

The need for continuing education programmes to be evaluated is widely recognized (Chambers 1988, Ferguson 1994, Parfitt 1986). Effective evaluation of educational programmes can inform decision-making, influence programme development and ultimately impact on nursing practice. Efforts to evaluate existing educational programmes in nursing have largely concentrated on basic nurse education courses (Chambers 1988). Strategies used to evaluate programmes of basic nursing can be incorporated into the evaluation of cancer courses, although there are specific issues to be considered because of the specialist nature of cancer nursing.

Much of the work on evaluating programmes of nursing is of an anecdotal nature and there is a lack of empirically based work considering nurses' perceptions of their continuing educational needs and benefits in terms of changes in knowledge and attitude (Ferguson 1994). Those who have conducted evaluative studies have tended to draw on aims, criteria and methods from sociology and/or general education or management rather than exploring the World Health Organization's curriculum aims of relevance to national healthcare needs and nurses' accountability to their clients (Chavasse 1994, Whiteley 1992).

Educational evaluation has evolved over a relatively short timespan and a number of different approaches have developed (Whiteley 1992). Evaluation is particularly valuable in the context of nursing education owing to the multifaceted nature of nursing education programmes. The complexity of educational evaluation has led to support for the principle of working within the framework of an accepted model of evaluation (Parfitt 1986, Whiteley 1992). There are several programme evaluation models available to guide the evaluation process. The general purposes of programme evaluation are to diagnose problems, weaknesses and strengths, and to consider the feasibility of a programme accomplishing its objectives. The importance of consistency in programme evaluation is widely recognized, as is the need for a systematic means of identifying a positive teaching and learning climate (Parfitt 1986, Wheeler 1988).

Professional accountability and financial demands on course organizers to demonstrate value for money have contributed to the growth of programme evaluation as a discipline (Chambers 1988). A number of other aims and purposes of curriculum evaluation have been described (Chavasse 1994). These include the need for validation where professional and academic bodies have their own criteria for accreditation, meeting objectives, curriculum improvement, and evaluation of innovations. In programme evaluation, as in other areas of nursing, it is the translation of theory into practice that causes greatest difficulty.

The value of adopting a holistic approach to the evaluation of educational programmes in order to obtain greater insight into specific courses is recognized (Parfitt 1986, Whiteley 1992). Models of evaluation appear to have evolved with reference to this change in focus. Early work on evaluation adopted a traditionally scientific approach and concentrated on measurement and prediction. Limitations of this approach in terms of its narrow perspective became apparent, and a shift in focus towards a more explorative stance occurred in which unintended or unexpected outcomes were also taken into consideration (Whitely 1992). In terms of programmes of nurse education, models of evaluation may serve as guidelines but evaluators need to adapt models for the purposes of their particular course (Watson & Herbener 1990). Illuminative evaluation based in description and interpretation incorporates the concepts of structure, process and outcome identified as key concepts in earlier models of evaluation (Whiteley 1992). Illuminative evaluation provides a general evaluation strategy that can be adapted to suit individual needs, and a number of those who have endeavoured to evaluate nursing courses have utilized this approach (Chambers 1988, Whiteley 1992).

Whitely (1992) applied the principles of structure, process and outcome in practice in her work evaluating continuing education courses in Scotland. Questionnaires and interviews were used as data collection tools. Information was sought on the structures available to provide and support the courses and on the processes by which the courses were planned, implemented and received. This was largely factual data, but information of a more qualitative nature was obtained when outcomes were considered in terms of the participants' perceptions of the courses. This sort of dual approach to course evaluation was seen as a useful means of investigation.

The evaluation of programme aims is implied in many studies but explicit matching of learning objectives and outcomes is unusual. Studies from the USA have placed a greater emphasis on whether or not a programme achieves its targets

(Pope 1992, Watson & Herbener 1990). The scarcity of outcome studies may be related to the complexity of measuring increases in knowledge and skills which are the intended product of nursing curricula. The identification of clearly defined objectives are crucial to the effective evaluation of educational programmes. According to Davies (1976), if an educational programme has no predetermined objectives it is equivalent to setting out on a journey without a map and will inevitably result in confusion, ambiguity and a breakdown in communication. This, in turn, will impede the evaluation of such programmes. Therefore, it is important to determine systematic evaluation of the project from the outset. As mentioned above, efforts to apply models of evaluation to practice have concentrated largely on basic nurse education programmes (Chambers 1988). Evaluating postbasic nursing courses is equally important for the development of continuing education.

Some of the components of educational programmes considered significant in terms of evaluation include conceptual framework, philosophy, programme goals, student characteristics, graduate performance, faculty and administrative expertise, and adequacy of resources (Chavasse 1994, Whiteley 1992). There are a number of specific factors to consider for evaluation within each component. The more tangible aspects of courses such as available facilities and course structure have been considered by those who have conducted programme evaluation (Chambers 1988, Whiteley 1992). Some of the less tangible aspects of courses are harder to evaluate and it is not always possible to evaluate all aspects of a programme simultaneously. Guidelines in the form of the EONS (1999) core curriculum may facilitate the construction of as broad a picture as possible in the case of education in cancer nursing.

The importance of a systematic approach to curriculum evaluation and compliance by those involved applies as much to cancer nurse education as to other nurse education programmes. In terms of evaluating cancer nurse education programmes, there are elements within the EONS (1999) core curriculum that guide this process.

Evaluation is most relevant when it builds upon and involves the people who are directly and indirectly affected by its results. To facilitate the future development of courses it is necessary to examine what is happening from the course members' frame of reference. Although increased knowledge and behavioural change are notoriously difficult to measure (Chavasse 1994), information on the subjective views of course organizers and participants can be gained through talking with them. Regarding course outcomes, further data in terms of efficiency and quality of nursing could be provided by patients (Watson & Herbener 1990). The provision of comprehensive quality care to patients with cancer is at the heart of educational courses in cancer nursing at basic and postbasic level and, therefore, should be being considered as an actual outcome of any educational programme.

EDUCATION IN RESPONSE TO HEALTHCARE POLICIES

If education is to be meaningful it must take cognisance of contemporary healthcare and the demands of health policy. Given the dynamic nature of healthcare in Europe at present, this task is not easily accomplished. Changing trends in healthcare and a move towards primary healthcare (Salvage 1997) need to be reflected in educational development. Those responsible for curriculum development must be aware of these factors whilst retaining a nursing ideology.

In Europe the notion of nursing as an ideology is difficult as the professional status of nursing remains an area of contention in many European countries.

In addition, in some countries nurses are still not responsible for developing educational programmes for nurses and it is deemed acceptable for physicians to determine nursing programmes. Although the World Bank (1993) has identified nurses as the most cost-effective resource for delivering high-quality public health, this is not always acknowledged by those responsible for managing this resource. This appears to be particularly apparent in central and eastern Europe and newly independent states, where there is evidence of failure to train staff adequately for their role or to deploy them effectively (Salvage 1997).

Whilst legal obligations in respect of nurse education have existed since 1977 in the European Union, some countries in this region remain unable or unwilling to comply with them (Salvage & Heijnen 1997). To facilitate education for practice it is claimed that nursing education should be supported at the highest levels so that programmes are (World Health Organization 1996):

1. based on the most recent assessment of the country's health needs and the need for nursing services
2. problem-based to promote skills of critical thinking and problem-solving
3. grounded in the philosophy of primary healthcare
4. based on current research in nursing practice
5. culturally appropriate
6. multidisciplinary, where appropriate, to encourage shared learning and greater understanding between professions.

The delivery of cancer care and the availability of education in this area varies greatly throughout the world. In Europe the diversity of education mirrors the international pattern. The Commission of the European Communities, through its Europe Against Cancer Programme, is addressing some of these variations with a number of recommendations. In their second action plan, the EC acknowledged that palliative cancer care provides extremely valuable support for patients for whom treatment has failed. It also recommended exchange of experience between member states for health professionals in the area of cancer care to improve training (European Commission 1990). This is reiterated in the third action plan for 1995–1999 (Commission of the European Communities 1995). Such recommendations allow policy-makers, as well as individual nurses, access to funds that would assist in the development of care for individuals requiring cancer care. The Europe Against Cancer Programme, however, is only one aspect of the EC's remit. The ratification of the Treaty on the European Union (Maastricht Treaty) offers nurses within the European Union the potential to play a leading role in shaping healthcare policy on a European and national level (Pritchard 1994). An important aspect of this responsibility includes promoting education. Educators in cancer care therefore have an opportunity to argue, within a legal structure, for the development of cancer services through education.

To improve the quality of healthcare provision, within the UK, the National Health Service (NHS) has undergone unprecedented changes and development. The new service is seeking to achieve greater response to individual needs, better value for money and an improvement in the quality of patient/client care. Nurses are clearly a major resource and the quality of their care will depend on the quality of their education (Department of Health 1994). The newly structured NHS expects that purchasers of healthcare will assess the total needs of the population they serve and in so doing will highlight the needs of cancer care provision. In order to meet those needs, an appropriately prepared and qualified workforce is required to be in place. Therefore, it is hoped that, in the future, education of nurses will be based upon regional needs analysis, demographic trends, skill-mix and financial resources.

The introduction of assessing the needs of communities and populations in relation to healthcare is likely to result in an increasing demand for appropriate cancer care and the provision of adequate and appropriately prepared staff. Currently in Britain, as in other European countries, the majority of patients with cancer receive treatment within a hospital setting. It is therefore essential that all levels of nursing staff can access relevant information and education regarding the care of patients with cancer and their significant others. However, the current shift of patient care from hospitals into the community requires that all nurses are prepared to be competent practitioners whatever the healthcare setting. This has implications for nursing education. It is essential that cancer care education prepares its students to be versatile and to practise competently in a variety of environments.

Whilst it is neither essential nor desirable, particularly in today's economic climate, that all nurses should be specialists in cancer care, it is important that cancer nursing education is available at various professional and academic levels and that those interested can access modules and programmes of study so that the public can expect a quality service irrespective of the setting and those who deliver it. In a number of developing countries active care of patients with chronic illnesses, such as cancer, is limited. Often care in this situation is, from the outset, palliative. We need therefore to ensure that through education we can address this phenomenon.

FUTURE DIRECTIONS

As both the science of cancer and the profession of nursing develops, education will be required that is both culturally and educationally sensitive. Education that meets the needs of patients is, of course, the ideal but educational programmes available today are rarely based on patient needs assessments. This is despite the fact that the most important outcome for any educational programme involving healthcare professionals is the impact it has on patient outcomes. There is a real urgency for developers of cancer nursing education programmes to acknowledge this and involve patients themselves at the developmental stage of curriculum development, thereby ensuring that their needs are addressed in the resulting curriculum. In addition, the evaluation of educational programmes rarely involves measurement of the impact of such programmes on patient care, resulting in a biased and somewhat secular view of the value of education in healthcare. The shift towards issues such as patient satisfaction and the increasing awareness of policy-makers regarding patient-lobbying groups should alert cancer nurse educators that the time is ripe for changing the focus of education from nurse to patient need. As well as this major attitudinal shift there are a number of other areas that will have a major impact on how nurses are educated in the future; these areas will now be addressed.

CONTINUING PROFESSIONAL EDUCATION

The concept of lifelong learning is thought to have emerged as a result of discussions during the United Nations International Education Year in 1970. The United Nations Educational, Scientific and Cultural Organization (UNESCO) adopted the notion in 1972 and presented it as a potential alternative to existing educational principles (Cross-Durrant 1991). The need for lifelong learning in nursing is paramount if nursing is to continue to assert itself as a profession. It has been claimed that the participation of nurses in continuing education has been accepted universally (Hagopian 1997). However, at a European level the acknowledgement of continuing professional education (CPE) for nurses has been slow and is often incorporated into continuing medical education.

As part of the European Year of Life Long Learning, the English National Board for Nursing, Midwifery and Health Visiting (ENB), supported by a grant from the

■ BOX 5.2 Principles of lifelong learning (adapted from ENB 1997)

- Should be practice led.
- Should be student centred.
- Wherever possible it should be evidence based.
- Responsive to needs of individual healthcare professionals.
- Ethical regard for the individual.
- Takes account of the context of practice.
- Equity in provision and opportunity.
- Identify those responsible for achieving lifelong learning.
- Lifelong learning will raise the expectations of nurses.
- Learning is facilitated by the dissemination of knowledge.
- Support the concept of collaborative approach to care delivery.

EC, organized a European symposium to contribute to a strategic approach to lifelong learning for nurses. Participants at the symposium (representing 12 European countries) identified the core principles underpinning lifelong learning (ENB 1997). These are presented in Box 5.2.

In addition to these principles, the development of CPE in cancer nursing at a European level will have to take account of a number of factors, including:

- access
- language
- culture
- professional status of nursing
- variability in pre-registration preparation.

None of the above is insurmountable and work is currently underway in Europe to consider the development of CPE. The Federation of European Cancer Societies, of which EONS is a member, has established a working party to consider the most effective way to promote and accredit CPE. Whilst work is at an early stage, there are clear plans to provide a structure to recognize educational programmes, and attempts to offer European credit points which will cross disciplines are being considered.*

MOBILITY OF NURSES

The delivery of nursing care varies throughout the European Union and it is likely that this has a direct correlation with the education that nurses in different countries receive and the quality and level of care they deliver. Through exchange programmes nurses have an opportunity to observe new practices and make comparisons with clinical practice in their own area. Nurses have limited opportunities to undertake such exchanges and facilitation through the Europe Against Cancer (EAC) programme would have the potential of encouraging harmonization of cancer nursing practice in the EU. Whilst for many nurses language remains a real barrier to mobility, the enlargement of the European Union may facilitate mobility, and in developing educational programmes it may be important to consider the possibility of cultural diversity.

*For more information contact the Federation of European Cancer Societies, 83 Avenue E Mounier, B-1200 Brussels, Belgium.

ACCREDITATION

At present there is no accreditation system for cancer nursing education operating at a European level. Individual countries are at varying stages of developing internal accreditation systems, with the UK probably the most advanced. The concept of accreditation criteria for educational programmes at a European level is complex and many of the factors described above in relation to CPE would have to be considered.

As a result of requests from many members, EONS has succeeded in developing such an accreditation system, which became operational in the autumn of 1999. For the first time in Europe this has provided educationalists with the opportunity to develop courses that will meet European standards. One of the major outcomes expected from this initiative will be a more consistent approach to cancer nurse education. This will offer both students and purchasers of education alike a clearer indication of the value of particular courses.

INFORMATION TECHNOLOGY

Information technology (IT) is affecting the way we live our everyday lives and is having an increasing impact in the delivery of healthcare. The development of nursing informatics as a subspecialty of nursing is testament to the potential such technology has for our practice. In many ways IT has been slow to infiltrate the world of nursing but there can be little doubt that its introduction will continue.

The educational opportunities afforded by IT are immense, not simply as a means to communicate to a wider audience but utilization of IT will also affect the traditional didactic methods of teaching, resulting in interactive student-directed learning. In 1988, Romano asserted that nursing informatics should be concerned with careful consideration of the nature of nursing and how nursing information is acquired, manipulated and used. Ten years later we are witnessing exactly this through the WISECARE project (Kearney et al 1998), which is utilizing IT to improve knowledge and knowledge-sharing between cancer nurses in Europe to enhance patient care. This is, after all, what education should be all about.

CONCLUSION

That education is vital to the development of cancer nursing cannot be disputed and indeed is inherent in each of the chapters presented in this book. However, this text is not attempting to be idealistic and this author acknowledges the difficulties experienced by many nurses wishing to access specialist cancer nursing education. The importance of an educated nursing workforce was identified by the EC more than 10 years ago, yet there remains, as in the provision of cancer care, variability in the provision of cancer nursing education.

It is likely that, at present, the majority of patients are receiving nursing care from nurses who have benefited from little, if any, specialist education in cancer nursing (Jodrell 1996). For example, in the UK there are some areas where less than 3% of nurses caring for patients with cancer have undertaken specialist education (Ferguson 1996), and following a review of cancer nursing education in Europe undertaken last year it is unlikely that this picture is atypical (Jodrell 1997). In fact, for many countries in Europe there are no educational opportunities for nurses to access even if they wanted to. This is despite available evidence which demonstrates that an educated nursing workforce improves the quality of care delivered to patients (Carr-Hill et al 1992) and that healthcare costs are reduced when appropriately qualified staff deliver nursing care (Sovie 1988). Therefore, if cancer nurses are to have a role in the new millennium, we must address the problem of educational provision and lobby both nationally and at a European level to change the disparity that exists.

REFERENCES

American Nurses Association 1980 Nursing a social policy statement. American Nurses Association, Kansas City

Carr-Hill R, Dixon P, Gibbs I et al 1992 Skill mix and the effectiveness of nursing care. Centre for Health Economics, University of York, York

Chambers M 1988 Curriculum evaluation: an approach towards appraising a post-basic psychiatric course. Journal of Advanced Nursing 13:330–340

Chavasse J 1994 Curriculum evaluation in nursing education: a review of the literature. Journal of Advanced Nursing 19:1024–1031

Commission of the European Communities 1986 'Europe Against Cancer' programme: proposal for a plan of action 1987–1989. Commission of the European Communities, Luxembourg

Commission of the European Communities 1995 Adopting an action plan 1995–1999 to combat cancer within the framework for action in the field of public health. Commission of the European Communities, Luxembourg

Copp K 1988 Education and training in cancer. A European perspective. Cancer Nursing 11:255–258

Corner J, Wilson-Barnett J 1992 The newly registered nurse and the cancer patient; an educational evaluation. International Journal of Nursing Studies 29:177–190

Corner J, Plant H, A'Hern R, Bailey C 1996 Non-pharmacological intervention for the management of breathlessness in lung cancer. Palliative Medicine 10:299–305

Cross-Durrant A 1991 Basil Yeaxlee and the origins of lifelong learning. In: Jarvis P (ed) Twentieth century thinkers in adult education. Routledge, New York, p 38

Davies I K 1976 Objectives in curriculum design. McGraw-Hill, New York

Davis B, Burnard P 1992 Academic levels in nursing. Journal of Advanced Nursing 17:1395–1400

Department of Health 1994 Nursing, midwifery and helath visiting. Statement of strategic intent. HMSO, London

English National Board 1997 Lifelong learning in Europe: developing a strategic approach. English National Board for Nursing, Midwifery and Health Visiting, London

European Commission 1989 Decision OJL 346.89/601/EEC. Official Journal of the European Commission, Luxembourg

European Commission 1990 Adopting a 1990–1994 action plan in the context of the Europe Against Cancer programme. Official Journal of the European Communities no. L 137/31, Luxembourg

European Oncology Nursing Society 1990 A core curriculum for a post basic course in cancer nursing. Cancer Nursing 13:123–128

European Oncology Nursing Society 1999 A care curriculum for a post-basic course in cancer nursing. 2nd edn. EONS, Brussels

Expert Advisory Group on Cancer 1995 A policy framework for commissioning cancer services. A report by the Expert Advisory Group on Cancer to the chief medical officers of England and Wales. Department of Health, London

Faithfull S 1995 'Just grin and bear it and hope it will go away': coping with urinary symptoms from pelvic radiotherapy. European Journal of Cancer Care 4:158–165

Ferguson A 1994 Evaluating the purpose and benefits of continuing education in nursing and the implications for the provision of continuing education for cancer nurses. Journal of Advanced Nursing 19:640–646

Ferguson A 1996 Workforce planning implications for nursing and professions allied to medicine of the Calman-Hine report. NHS Executive, Northern and Yorkshire, England

Hagopian G 1997 Advancing cancer nursing through nursing education. In: Groenwald S, Frogge M, Goodman M, Henke Yarbro C (eds) Cancer nursing: principles and practice, 4th edn. Jones & Bartlett, London, pp 1666–1678

Hamric A B 1995 Advanced practice: the future is now. Oncology Nursing Forum 22(3):547–553

James N D, Gurrero D, Brada M 1994 Who should follow up cancer patients? Nurse specialist based outpatient care and the introduction of a phone clinic system. Clinical Oncology 6:283–287

Jodrell N 1996 Cancer nursing services in Scotland: are we ready to meet the challenge? NT Research 1(5):375–380

Jodrell N 1997 An assessment of the activities in the area of training in oncology for nurses. Europe Against Cancer programme, project no. 96/CAN/47281. European Commission, Luxembourg

Kearney N, Campbell S, Sermeus W 1998 Practising for the future: utilising information technology in cancer nursing practice. European Journal of Oncology Nursing 2(3):169–175

Kelly B 1991 The professional values of English nursing undergraduates. Journal of Advanced Nursing 16:867–872

Knowles G, Kearney N 1998 Advancing cancer nursing practice in Europe: an overview. European Journal of Oncology Nursing 2(3):156–161

Lake T, Jenkins J 1993 Cancer chemotherapy: clinical trials. Cancer Nursing 16(6):186–197

Lawson N 1993 Meeting the needs of patients with cancer. Cancer Relief Macmillan Fund, Edinburgh

McArdle J M C, George W D, McArdle C S et al 1996 Psychological support for patients undergoing breast cancer surgery: a randomised study. British Medical Journal 312:813–816

Mackintosh C, Bowles S 1997 Evaluation of a nurse-led acute pain service. Can clinical nurse specialists make a difference? Journal of Advanced Nursing 25:30–37

McVie G 1996 Current areas of treatment. Seminars in Oncology 23(supp1):1–3

Maguire P, Tait Brooke M A et al 1980 Effect of counselling on the psychiatric morbidity associated with mastectomy. British Medical Journal 281:1454–1455

Mallows C et al 1990 An evaluation of nurse specialists diabetic clinics. Practical Diabetes 7:21–23

O'Brian et al 1991 Urinary incontinence: prevalence, need for treatment and effectiveness of intervention by nurse. British Medical Journal 303:1308–1311

Parfitt B 1986 Steps in evaluating a programme of nurse education. Nurse Education Today, 6:166–171

Palsson B E, Norberg A 1995 Breast cancer patients' experiences of nursing care with the focus on emotional support: the implementation of a nursing intervention. Journal of Advanced Nursing 21:277–285

Pfister-Minogue K 1993 Enhancing patient compliance: a guide for nurses. To increase their patients' compliance with health recommendations nurse need a framework. Geriatric Nursing 14(13):124–132

Preston N 1995 New strategies for the management of malignant ascites. European Journal of Cancer Care 4:178–183

Pope S 1992 Fundamentals for a new concept of oncology nursing in the professional education program. Cancer Nursing 15(2):137–147

Pritchard P 1994 The Maastricht Treaty: setting a healthcare agenda for Europe. European Journal of Cancer Care 3:6–11

Rich S E 1993 Tamoxifen and breast cancer – from palliation to prevention. Cancer Nursing 16(5): 341–346

Romano C 1988 Preparing nurses for the development and implementation of information systems. In: Peterson H, Gerdin-Jegler U (eds) Preparing nurses for using information systems: recommended informatics competencies. National League for Nursing, New York, p 83

Rosenthal D S 1998 Changing trends. CA: A Cancer Journal for Clinicians 48:3–4

Royal College of Nursing Cancer Nursing Society 1996a A structure for cancer nursing services. Royal College of Nursing, London

Royal College of Nursing Cancer Nursing Society 1966b Guidelines for good practice in cancer nursing education. Royal College of Nursing, London

Salvage J 1997. In: Salvage & Heijnens (eds) Nursing in Europe: a resource for better health. WHO Regional Publications, European Series no. 74. WHO, Geneva, p 5

Salvage J, Heijnen S 1997 Nursing and midwifery in Europe. In: Salvage J, Serge (eds) Nursing in Europe: a resource for better health. WHO Regional Publications, European Series no. 74. WHO, Geneva, p 21

Sneddon M 1992 Continuing education in palliative care nursing: an evaluation of perceived outcome and factors influencing application of learning. MSc thesis, University of Glasgow, Glasgow

Sovie M D 1988 Variable costs of nursing care in hospitals. Annual Review of Nursing Research 6

Standing Committee of Nurses of the European Union 1995 Report: workshop on cancer nursing in basic nurse education. Standing Committee of Nurses of the European Union, Brussels

United Kingdom Central Council for Nursing, Midwifery and Health Visiting 1994 The future of professional practice – the council's standards for education and practice following registration. UKCC, London

Wade B 1990 Colostomy patients' psychological adjustment. Journal of Advanced Nursing 15:1297–1304

Watson J, Herbener D 1990 Programme evaluation in nursing education: the state of the art. Journal of Advanced Nursing 15:316–323

Watson M, Denton S, Baum M, Greer S, 1988 Counselling breast cancer patients: a specialist nurse service. Counselling Psychology Quarterly 1:25–35

Wheeler H 1988 Evaluating study modules in basic nurse education programmes. Nurse Education Today 8:77–84

Whiteley S 1992 Evaluation of nursing-education programmes – theory and practice. International Journal of Nursing Studies 29:315–323

Wilkinson S 1986 The satisfactions and stresses experienced of nursing cancer patients. MSc thesis, University of Manchester, Manchester

Wilkinson S 1991 Factors which influence how nurses communicate with cancer patients. Journal of Advanced Nursing 16:677–688

World Bank 1993 Investing in health; the World Bank development report. The World Bank, New York

World Health Organization 1996 Nursing practice. Report of a WHO expert committee. WHO Technical Report series no. 860. WHO, Geneva

Wouters B 1994 Teaching palliative care: a challenge to nursing trainers. European Journal of Palliative Care 1:178–183

Yeaxlee B A 1929 Lifelong education. Cassell, London

Nursing research in cancer care

Alison Richardson   Paola Di Giulio   Derek Waddell

CHAPTER 6

INTRODUCTION

The importance of research in cancer care has long been recognized and accepted by nurses involved in this field (European Oncology Nursing Society 1992). Research can provide us with one element of the critical knowledge base concerned with the care of patients with cancer, complementing that contributed by tradition and ritual, authority, experience and intuition. Research should underpin the science of cancer nursing care, and the role of research in the development of a body of knowledge for the education, practice and management of our discipline should be examined continually.

Oberst (1978) described the importance of cancer nursing research over two decades ago when she remarked that 'the challenges for nurses working in the rapidly changing milieu of cancer care are enormous. New treatment regimes continually force re-examination of old assumptions about patients' needs, and demand the development of new strategies for effective nursing care' (p. 281). In order that we achieve research-based cancer nursing practice, a number of strategies are required; these include those that improve knowledge, those that encourage implementation of research findings in practice and those that relate to the conduct of new research in clinical practice. Hence, the focus of this chapter will be on the role of the cancer nurse in the development, implementation and application of cancer nursing research. It will acknowledge that the conduct of independent nursing research is only one dimension of research in cancer nursing and thus will also examine the role of nurses working within the context of the organization and conduct of clinical trials. The resources available to support research related to the areas of interest to cancer nurses will be detailed.

Research carried out by, and in collaboration with, nurses involved in cancer care in Europe is not prolific. It is a challenging area, and one in which European nurses still need a large degree of help in order to develop an appropriate level of expertise (Arrigo 1991). This chapter will, in part, rehearse and extend many of the issues raised by educators, researchers, managers and practising cancer nurses in relation to the best means of meeting the research needs of European cancer nurses.

THE SCOPE OF CANCER NURSING RESEARCH

Several published papers provide concise summaries of early and more current research which relates to the specialty, principally relating to developments in the USA, Canada and the UK (Degner 1984, Fernsler, Holcombe & Pulliam 1984, Grant & Padilla 1983, McCorkle & Lewis 1980, Padilla 1990, Richardson & Wilson-Barnet 1995). More recently, a meta-analysis of cancer nursing research was reported by Smith & Stullenberger (1995). This was conducted with the purpose of describing 10 years of patient-related oncology nursing research in the USA. It might be illuminating, if somewhat more difficult, to conduct such an exercise within a European or international context.

In addition to historical and contemporary reviews of research in the specialty, there are a growing number of cancer nursing research reviews that have focused on a variety of topics deemed of importance to nurses working in the field of cancer care. The conduct of such reviews is an important vehicle through which to access the steady accumulation of evidence generated through research, whether it be exploratory, descriptive, correlational, comparative or experimental in nature. Although research reviews of the type noted previously add to the body of knowledge, meta-analyses are regarded as superior when attempting to combine the results of similar studies to examine the strength of research findings in the chosen area, due to rigorous adherence to a defined protocol and utilization of reliable data-collection instruments. Smith, Holcombe & Stullenberger (1994) conducted such an analysis of symptom management intervention studies. However, presently, meta-analyses, by their very nature, only incorporate studies that are experimental in nature.

Nursing research in cancer care is concerned with both the impact of the disease and its treatment on the patient and family and the efficacy of nursing care in both alleviating and ameliorating disease or treatment-induced problems (Corner 1993). Cancer nursing care offers researchers an opportunity to study diverse problems in a natural setting, a setting in which it is sometimes neither feasible nor desirable to conduct controlled experiments. Hence, to place sole value on work that adopts an experimental or quasi-experimental approach is to deny the equally important contribution that studies which have their roots in either survey methodology or the qualitative paradigms make to the growth of the knowledge-base of cancer nursing. In those areas where little is known about a problem area, it is prudent to undertake well-designed exploratory–descriptive studies in which the researcher documents systematically the issues, concepts, ideas or phenomena under study. As more is known, a comparative or correlational design (often referred to as survey designs) may be more appropriate. Quasi-experimental and experimental designs have a tendency to be used when much is known about a problem area and the variables that influence it. A further type of research, the methodological study, is used to develop and test data collection instruments. This is a previously neglected but presently evolving area of nursing research generally, and this holds true in the field of nursing research in cancer care.

Another means of gaining an impression, particularly of areas that should receive attention in future research investigations, can be obtained through reference to national surveys of research priorities. Such priority-setting exercises are increasingly being seen as a means to identify systematically where investment might be potentially made, in terms of both financial resources and intellect. There have been a number of surveys of priorities for cancer nursing research reported in the literature since 1978 when Oberst first published a Delphi survey. Subsequently, priority surveys have been conducted by national nursing organizations and consortiums of researchers, for example by the Canadian Consortium (Western Consortium for Cancer Nursing Research 1987), and on a regular basis by the Research Committee of the US Oncology Nursing Society (Funkhouser & Grant 1989, Grant & Stromborg 1981, McGuire, Frank-Stromborg & Varricchio 1985, Mooney et al 1991, Stetz et al 1995). Until recently, there were no comparative data with which to compare the priorities articulated by practising Canadian and US cancer nurses and their counterparts in Europe. However, work by the Nursing Research Special Interest group of the Dutch Oncology Nursing Society (Nieweg et al 1996) now makes a tentative comparison possible (Table 6.1). The results reveal that it would not be wise to assert that priorities identified through US surveys relate to the situation in Europe. This was not the finding when results were compared between the US and Canada (Western Consortium for Cancer Nursing Research 1987). Top-ranked priorities were essentially the same.

Table 6.1 Comparison of the 1994 US Oncology Nursing Society and 1995 Dutch Oncology Nursing Society research priorities

US Oncology Nursing Society		Dutch Oncology Nursing Society	
Category	Rank	Category	Rank
Symptom management	1	Psychosocial aspects of care	1
Psychosocial aspects of care	2	Continuum of care	2
Health promotion behaviours	3	Care delivery issues	3
Treatment decision-making	4	Treatment decision-making	3
Care delivery issues	4	Symptom management	4
Continuum of care	5	Health promotion behaviours	5
Special population	6	Special population	6

The lack of coherence in the focus of investigations between the USA and Europe has been noted previously by Corner (1997). She regards that the reviews previously cited do not include important areas being pursued by European cancer nurses, either singularly or collectively, such as dyspnoea, fatigue, lymphoedema, and the management of ascites, fungating wounds and symptoms that result from radiotherapy. This is not surprising since the reviews focus on published sources which almost exclusively cite work that is American in origin, dictated by the nature of the review process adopted.

CURRENT STATUS OF RESEARCH IN EUROPE

One reason, amongst many, that might account for the lack of similarity between the ranked priorities of European and US cancer nurses is perhaps related to the undoubted differences that exist in the stage of development of cancer nursing research that has been reached by the two continents. It is widely acknowledged across many European countries that research in this area is in its infancy. In order to ascertain the current status of cancer nursing research in Europe, a brief survey was conducted in March 1997, based in some respects on a survey conducted by the International Society of Nurses in Cancer Care (Fitch 1996). The survey was sent to a representative of each national cancer nursing organization. Twenty-three survey questionnaires were distributed and these focused on such aspects as access to cancer nursing research expertise, funding for conducting nursing research and for studying about nursing research and current areas of research in cancer nursing, both independent and as part of a PhD programme. Thirteen were returned.

The responses provide us with information, albeit limited, on the current status of cancer nursing research in the countries in question. Access to cancer nursing research expertise was considered to be somewhat of a problem by the majority of respondents (n = 6), whereas access to funding, both to conduct and to study about nursing research, was an issue of greater concern, being judged to be a major problem by seven of the 13 respondents. Methods of funding for conducting and studying in relation to nursing research varied; the responses are summarized in Table 6.2.

Just under half of the countries had candidates registered for the degree of PhD in an area related to cancer nursing. Topics included symptom management, care delivery and psychosocial aspects of care.

Obviously, the responses do not equate with the sum total of research activity in the area of cancer nursing in Europe today. It must be acknowledged that the

Table 6.2 Sources of funding identified for the conduct and study of nursing research

Source of funding category	Stated no. supporting the conduct of research	Stated no. supporting study about nursing research
Government (central)	2	3
Government (local or regional)	1	1
Pharmaceutical industry	6	2
National cancer nursing organizations	2	–
National nursing organizations	2	3
Cancer foundations and charities	7	4
Hospital	2	3
University scholarships	1	1
Research councils (national and European)	2	–
Healthcare foundations and charities	4	2

representatives who completed the questionnaires may not have been in the best position to report on the issues raised. Indeed, some admitted that, for example, they were aware of a number of PhD candidates and independent researchers, but could not detail their names and areas of research. This information was obviously not easy to come by and perhaps points to the fact that, in order to foster networking and collaboration, an important first step is to learn who is engaged in cancer nursing research and the focus of such work. However, it can probably be stated with some level of certainty that activity in relation to research in areas of interest to cancer nursing is patchy in Europe, as are the resources to support both the conduct and study of research.

This mirrors the picture found in relation to nursing research generally in Europe. An Expert Committee on Nursing Research recently published a report and recommendations on nursing research in which it was stated that 'while nursing service and education have long traditions, investments in nursing research was in many countries sporadic, limited or even non-existent' (European Health Committee 1996, p. 9). Nursing research in Europe is still in an early stage of development (Tierney 1994), although beginning to develop at a steady pace, and recommendations have recently been made regarding the establishment of a model strategy for its development (European Health Committee 1996). Key considerations include:

- The development of structure and organization
- Measures to ensure the integration of research and practice
- Education in the skills required for the conduct of nursing research
- Provision of funds for research and research education
- Means to encourage and promote collaboration between countries.

STRATEGIC DEVELOPMENT

There has been frequent acknowledgement that we should pay attention to the development of research along the lines set out in the model above. A number of accounts have appeared that provide an analysis of the many factors that are recognized as obstacles to realizing the measured development of cancer nursing research in Europe (Arrigo 1991, Corner 1991, European Health Committee 1996, Payne 1993, Tierney 1997). These will be referred to in the discussion that follows.

Education and training

There is recognition that facilities to enable nurses across Europe to acquire the knowledge and skills required to initiate, implement and evaluate valid and reliable research are vital to ensuring a comprehensive programme of cancer nursing research. Nursing needs to remain realistic about both the desirability and the possibility of nurses becoming involved in research activity. There are various levels of research knowledge required to increase the body of knowledge in cancer nursing and these are often equated with different levels of educational preparation, i.e. diploma, degree, master's and doctorate level (European Health Committee 1996, McGuire & Harwood 1989, Mooney & Haberman 1996). In 1992, the European Oncology Nursing Society (EONS), in collaboration with representatives from major cancer nursing organizations involved in research in Europe, prepared a core curriculum for use throughout Europe on the topic of research for nurses in cancer care (see Box 6.1).

Levels of involvement in research can be seen as a continuum: at one end is the nurse engaged in delivering care that is research based, and at the other is the nurse in a position to be able to lead independent research. However, it would be short-sighted to assert that one holds a position of superiority over the other, and they are certainly not mutually exclusive, although there is often such a risk when levels of research involvement are equated with levels of educational preparation. All nurses have a responsibility to continually develop the scientific body of knowledge to guide cancer nursing practice; indeed, specialist knowledge and experience in cancer care are a prerequisite when developing relevant research questions. This includes nurses involved in clinical practice, education, research and management, and will increasingly include those in roles that have been instigated to help bridge the gap between research, practice and education (Graydon et al 1993). However, such models can provide the basis for planning research involvement and the design of programmes of education to support such involvement. This is vital if nurses are to participate in the research process to advance the clinical practice of cancer nursing.

As Mooney & Haberman (1996) point out, responsibilities are not necessarily distinct. Experience, interest and research training of the particular nurse may increase the degree of research involvement. The distinction made by the Workgroup of European Nurse Researchers (WENR) between research education and research training (Tierney 1997), which describes the former as concerned with the development of research appreciation skills in all nurses, and the latter as the formal preparation of nurses as researchers, is a helpful one.

Fostering research-based practice

Through the articulation of different levels of involvement in research there is an acknowledgement that not every nurse can, or should, be a researcher. To direct a research project requires a catalogue of specialist knowledge and skills. However, there are a number of research-related roles that are important for cancer nurses to embrace. If nurses working in the field of cancer care fail to adopt such roles, the results of research will not find their way into clinical practice. Fitch & Thompson (1996) have described these as Consumer, Facilitator, Contributor and Advocate.

Acting in the role of research Consumer principally involves being aware of research that has been conducted in the field and using it appropriately in practice. Adopting the role of Facilitator requires assisting others in the conduct of research and could potentially include, for example, identifying the best means of

---

■ BOX 6.1 Objectives of the core curriculum on research for nurses in cancer care

The core curriculum has three central components:
1. An introduction to research in nursing
2. The research process
3. Issues in nursing research.

An introduction to research in nursing

- To develop understanding of research as a systematic approach to enquiry for the purpose of developing new knowledge; and the relationship of research to theory and knowledge about clinical practice
- To discuss different research approaches and philosophical traditions
- To explore ethical and professional issues in nursing research
- To appreciate the extent to which nursing has developed its own scientific knowledge-base derived from nursing research studies.

The research process

- To appreciate the importance of examining previous literature before designing a research study
- To develop skills in systematic literature search
- To develop skills in critical appraisal of published research studies
- To develop understanding of each of the steps of the research process
- To develop skills in the techniques of data collection and analysis
- To develop confidence in undertaking each of the steps in the research process
- To develop skills in writing research proposals and reports.

Issues in nursing research

- To reflect on the role of nurses in research, both in nursing and in the wider health-care field
- To appreciate the need for research supervision and peer support while undertaking research
- To examine the difficulties and constraints in undertaking research and implementing research findings
- To evaluate published research
- To discuss political and funding issues in relation to nursing research.

From European Oncology Nursing Society (1992), with permission

---

approaching potential research subjects in a clinical area, to delivering an intervention as dictated in a research protocol. When practising nurses raise ideas for research questions with investigators, they play a valuable role as Contributor and, because of the profound effect of cancer and cancer treatment on the patient, cancer nursing care has provided a rich source of questions and problems for nursing research investigators. Acting in the capacity of research Advocate involves being an advocate both with respect to ensuring that practice is, as far as possible, based on research, and for subjects involved in a research study.

Increasingly our attentions are being turned to the effective utilization of the body of research-based knowledge that is already in existence, and the barriers that must be overcome to achieve this, whilst not detracting from the relentless pursuit for new knowledge which results from the conduct of scientific investigations. Whilst focusing on the discrete area of palliative care, rather than cancer care *per se*, a Delphi survey conducted by Cawley & Webber (1995), with the intent of determining the clinical research priorities, identified items for research for which there were frequently existing research findings. Oberst (1978), in an earlier survey devoted to cancer nurses' priorities, found a similar pattern. Such surveys serve to highlight the pressing need to find more effective ways of disseminating relevant research findings, not just to nurses, but to the entire healthcare community. With the accumulation of collections of studies and the application of meta-analytic techniques, it has become possible to focus attention on transforming credible findings into clinical protocols and guidelines. Unfortunately, research utilization is an active process for which the majority of nurses have not been prepared.

The extent of the barriers perceived both by oncology staff nurses and nurse managers/clinical nurse specialists to research utilization have recently been described by Rutledge et al (1998), using the previously developed Barriers Scale of Funk et al (1991). This scale includes potential barriers to research utilization:

1. Characteristics of the adopter (the nurse) of the innovation, such as nurse's value of research and perceived need for change
2. Characteristics of the organization, such as insufficient time or lack of cooperation
3. Characteristics of the innovation (research) itself such as inadequate research and conflicting findings
4. Characteristics of the communication of the innovation such as unclear implications for practice.

Nurses are asked to rate 28 items based on the degree to which they perceive them to be barriers. In the group of nurses surveyed, organizational, research and communication barriers persist as impediments to research utilization, and as a group these nurses responded similarly to other nurse samples who have completed the scale (as described by Funk, Tonquist & Champagne 1995).

Efforts to decrease known barriers will require changes for nurses in all roles, whether it be practice, education or research management. As yet, however, there is little published literature to indicate the most effective routes to pursue in the development and implementation of research utilization programmes in cancer care settings, including the processes involved and outcomes that might be predicted, against which the success of such ventures can be evaluated. An exception to this was a programme developed at a nursing department of a comprehensive cancer centre in the US (McGuire, Walczak & Krumm 1994). This programme provided many insights into the challenges of incorporating research findings into clinical practice and alludes to the diffuse and complex nature of research utilization. It demonstrated the usefulness of adopting a structured model, in this case the Stetler–Marram Model of Research Utilization (Stetler 1994), through which to focus on the phases through which it is necessary to progress in order to ensure effective research utilization.

It is important that nurses actively seek ways of acquiring the skills needed to read research papers, review and discuss these for applicability to practice, and evaluate recommendations for use in practice. Educators must include as part of their remit the development of innovative courses concerned with the utilization and conduct of research at all levels of education, rather than maintaining the current emphasis in many programmes on its conduct. They have a responsibility to act in the capacity of role model and mentor, inspiring students into valuing evidence-based practice, for example through the use of research in teaching about the practice of cancer nursing. Managers need constantly to strive to create a practice environment that values the importance of research in addressing patient care problems, demonstrating nursing and patient outcomes, and evaluating costs and quality issues.

Inevitably, research utilization efforts sanctioned by management have the greatest chance of success, and the role of management should be increasingly recognized in providing visible support for, and eliminating the barriers to, staff participation. Researchers must begin to play a central role in this process. This might be realized through studying problems that inform clinical practice decision-making and through the conduct of studies and testing interventions that can be transferred into clinical practice. Advances in cancer nursing and improvements in the quality of patient care will be attained more rapidly through the utilization of findings and the application of the research process to new approaches to patient care.

Dissemination

As stated above, patient care could be improved substantially by developing existing resources in cancer nursing research and in nursing generally. Historically, nurse researchers have focused primarily on the conduct of studies, rather than transforming research findings into a form of information useful to clinical practice. However, as Tierney (1997) states, 'research activity is, of course, of no value at all if its results are not properly disseminated to those who will make use of its findings' (p. 80). Researchers have an obligation to communicate the results of a study, the findings relevant to practice, and implications for further research. Dissemination is an intrinsic component of the research utilization process, and issues that need to be addressed to facilitate this process include consideration of who should disseminate findings, the manner in which it should be done, and finally the locations chosen to undertake dissemination.

Scientific meetings and conferences of a regional, national, European or international nature are regarded as valuable, albeit traditional, vehicles through which to pursue research dissemination. The value of these cannot be underestimated, especially when simultaneous translation is available, as language is a major barrier to research dissemination in Europe. In addition, activities can be planned with the explicit purpose of bringing clinical nurses into close contact with researchers, creating an ideal medium through which to cultivate collaboration.

Publication remains the main medium for research dissemination, and a number of peer-reviewed international and European journals are devoted to the discipline of cancer nursing. For example, *Cancer Nursing* (J B Lippincott) is the official publication of the International Society of Nurses in Cancer Care. However, such publications frequently appear only in the English language, thereby producing an insurmountable barrier to the vast majority of European cancer nurses. The arrival of the *European Journal of Oncology Nursing* (Churchill Livingstone), the official peer-reviewed journal of EONS, in which abstracts will appear in two European languages in addition to English, is expected to make a significant contribution to helping to solve this daunting issue, so intrinsically linked to that of dissemination. Similarly, *Oncology Nurses Today*, a pan-European magazine-type publication, appears in no fewer than nine languages. The availability of a number of different publications is likely to increase the chances of individual nurses locating a style of presentation which they find both friendly and understandable. Many clinical journals have altered the presentation of descriptions of research studies to enhance readability, and now place differing levels of emphasis on the interpretation of research findings and practice implications.

Guidelines developed by careful evaluation of available evidence with input from practitioners help to encourage and direct evidence-based and good clinical practice. Integrative literature reviews which elucidate practice implications are another valuable approach. START, an acronym for State of the Art Oncology in Europe, is a project currently underway which is concerned with creating an evidence-based knowledge instrument on the state-of-the-art treatment of malignant tumours and other topics of clinical importance to cancer care. Its construction and updating involves almost 200 leading European oncologists and is coordinated by a taskforce of oncologists based at the Instuto Nazionale dei Tumori and at the European Institute of Oncology in Milan. The first chapters are now accessible through the Internet at the website http://www.oncoweb.com/START, and feedback opportunities will be offered by e-mail to allow communication between the project team and healthcare professionals involved in cancer care who consult the database. It has been recognized that enhanced use of information technology may help enable dissemination of integrative reviews, research-based protocols and clinical guidelines (Crane 1995). Outcome indicators need to be identified to enable the effectiveness of such initiatives to be audited.

The Cochrane Centre in Oxford, UK, has made significant progress in developing a role in providing, maintaining and disseminating systematic reviews of reliable evidence from around the world about the effects of individual healthcare interventions. Each reviewer in the Cochrane Collaboration is a member of a review group sharing an interest in a particular topic, coordinated by an editorial team. The reviews are heavily dependent on the electronic transfer of information, and are disseminated both online (www.update-software.com/ccweb/cochrane/cdsr.htm) and by CD-ROM.

Coordination, cooperation and collaboration

Presently, in individual countries across Europe and at an international level, there is little coordination of research activity. Corner (1993) considered that this may undermine the development of a coherent body of knowledge that can be developed to influence and direct practice. In response to this, a group of nurses active in cancer research met to identify strategies for promoting research activity and to develop a framework for the development of nursing research in cancer care. Although developed as a reaction to the picture in the UK, Corner (1993) acknowledged that such a strategy could be developed across Europe. The framework outlined centres on identifying mechanisms by which research activity can be promoted, and includes the following (Corner 1993, p. 114):

- Identifying the characteristic features of nursing research in cancer care
- Agreeing on key areas of focus for research toward which resources might be directed
- Identifying the most appropriate mechanisms for building programmes of research
- Identifying how best to create milieus conducive to the development of cancer nurse researchers.

To move the cancer nursing research agenda forward in Europe, it is essential to identify both the priority areas for research and the human capacity to conduct it. This means identifying existing centres that have the necessary facilities and capabilities, and establishing schemes to train and develop researchers. There are a number of different settings in Europe in which cancer nursing research is conducted on a scale beyond that of isolated single studies. They vary widely in structure and in the personnel involved, and include clusters of cancer nurse researchers working within departments of nursing in universities, university-based centres (for example, at the Catholic University in Leuven, Belgium), practice-based units, such as the Worthing Nursing Development Unit based at Worthing and

Southlands Hospital in the UK, and centres funded by charitable research money. An example of the latter is the Macmillan Practice Development Unit based at the Centre for Cancer and Palliative Care at the Institute of Cancer Research in London. Excellent work has been done by individuals and by a small number of teams, but this needs to be further developed and supported.

There are many potential advantages and disadvantages to different organizational approaches that may be adopted to support cancer nursing research. Such approaches might include the development of self-contained units dedicated to cancer nursing research or a variety of collaborations within existing research units. One constructive way forward might be through the development of multidisciplinary teams to encourage collaboration between experienced and novice researchers, promoting access to varied skills, experience and resources. There is a need to build up a critical mass of cancer nursing research in a number of institutions which can also provide support for individual research talent. Without this, cancer nursing will fare badly in competition for funds, and potential researchers will become discouraged. However, it is acknowledged that there are powerful structural and organizational reasons that mitigate against the development of cancer nursing research (Payne 1993), and it will require a great deal of determination and some semblance of political awareness to make progress in implementing any such framework.

An important step in achieving a coordinated European approach to cancer nursing research is learning who is engaged in cancer nursing research in Europe. This would aid the identification of partners able to engage in collaborative research ventures and pinpoint those able to act in the capacity of a resource, from whom individuals could seek mutual support and advice while involved in research. EONS has articulated its role in relation to research and this focuses on identifying and building on the body of knowledge specific to cancer nursing and encouraging the development of, and participation in, collaborative research. With this in mind, a directory of expert nurses involved in education, practice and research is in the process of being established by EONS. There should be a focus on what can best be accomplished within, and through, the European community of nurses involved in cancer care. Through the World Wide Web there are almost limitless possibilities to network such a database with similar databases being established around the world. Of particular note is the current initiative of the International Society of Nurses in Cancer Care concerned with identifying nursing research studies in which cancer is a major element through establishing a Directory of Nurse Researchers in Oncology.

One of the criticisms levelled at nursing research in cancer care is that studies continue to recruit small samples; are largely descriptive in nature; rarely study any single subject in depth; or involve replication or the testing of interventions using traditional clinical research designs (Smith & Stullenberger 1995). It has been suggested that in order to increase the productivity of individual studies we must expend a considerable amount of effort on designing and conducting collaborative projects (Oberst 1979). This should include both intranursing and interdisciplinary collaborative research. The benefits of collaborative efforts are tremendous and include the ability to address complex patient care problems, the generation of clinically relevant research, entry into acute and chronic care settings, and the acquisition of large sample sizes from which results may be generalizable (Stone 1991). To this end, progress has already been made in a number of areas.

A pan-European survey funded through an educational grant from a pharmaceutical company was recently conducted to identify the current communication channels between patients with cancer and their healthcare teams, and highlighted the key aspects required to achieve effective communication (Denton 1996). The survey was developed and conducted by a multidisciplinary Working Group on

Living with Advanced Breast Cancer Hormone Treatment. The Checklist for Patients on Endocrine Therapy (C-PET) was developed as a result of the need identified in the pan-European survey, which offers healthcare professionals the means of improving communication (Hopwood 1996).

In the area of fatigue, the Action on Fatigue programme, again funded by a pharmaceutical company, has made possible the development of a collaborative nursing research initiative across Europe. The management of fatigue, alongside oral care, is one of the priorities of care identified through the EC funded WISECARE project (Workflow Information Systems for European Nursing project) (Jodrell 1996). This collaborative project involving five demonstration sites across Europe will provide a model through which to monitor outcomes as well as the cost of services to patients in relation to these two care priorities. This will be achieved through the development of a workflow information model enabling the systematic exploitation of electronic clinical nursing data sets. If successful, this project will prove to be a landmark in terms of cancer nurses' attempts to harmonize the measurement of outcomes in Europe. The project provides for the dissemination of state-of-the-art European guidelines and protocols, and will provide tools to compare actual practice with benchmarks.

CLINICAL TRIALS AND CANCER NURSING RESEARCH

Potentially, the nurse may hold several but interrelated roles in the implementation of research related to patients with cancer. As a practising cancer nurse, this may include being a member, formal or informal, of a research team conducting the research. Another role may be the initiation of a study, known as companion studies, alongside a medical protocol. Obviously, the most rewarding role is when the nurse acts in the capacity of principal investigator, initiating the study, writing the proposal, recruiting subjects and evaluating the results.

What is a clinical trial?

A clinical trial is a research study conducted in human beings and designed to answer specific questions using scientifically controlled methods. Results of clinical trials are widely recognized as contributing to a sound knowledge-base for the treatment of various illnesses and providing the only scientifically reliable evidence on which recommendations for treatments should be established (Di Giulio et al 1996). Each study is outlined in a document called a protocol, where objectives of the study are described, details on the specific treatment to be administered are provided, and criteria for selecting the patients, treatment regimens, data collection, toxicity reporting, response determinations, regulatory requirements and procedures necessary for analysis of the results are listed (Cassidy & McFarlane 1991). The main components of a clinical study protocol are described in Box 6.2. All clinical trials are conducted according to a set of rules identified as Good Clinical Practices (GCPs). GCPs are a set of guidelines by which clinical trials are designed, implemented and reported, so that there is assurance that data are credible and that the rights, integrity and confidentiality of subjects are protected (see Box 6.3).

Clinical trials are mainly implemented to evaluate the efficacy of new therapies and treatments and their side-effects. Not all cancer clinical trials involve the use of chemotherapeutic agents: trials may also investigate the use and effectiveness of other types of treatments, such as radiation therapy, surgical interventions,

■ BOX 6.2   Essential components of a study protocol

Objectives of the study	Specific questions or hypothesis to be answered upon completion of the study. There may be one or more complementary objectives.
Scientific background and study rationale	The rationale of the study and its objectives should be clear and based on analysis of published literature.
Patient selection criteria	The criteria that define which patients will participate in the study and/or be excluded.
Pharmaceutical information	Information on the drug, stability, toxicities, etc.
Study design	The methodology used to achieve the aims of the study. A schematic diagram should be used in more complicated trial designs to illustrate the patients' course of treatment. The design of a phase I trial involves the selection of a drug dose (as selected from toxicological studies) and sequential dose escalations in a limited group of patients, until the maximum tolerated dose is achieved. Phase II studies start from a stated dose and evaluate cumulative and delayed toxicity. Phase III studies are randomised clinical trials.
Treatment plan	Treatments to be administered, dosages, administration times.
Toxicity evaluation criteria	The instrument criteria to assess severity of side-effects.
Dose adjustment plan	Changes in drug dosages according to patients' reactions.
Required study parameters for patient monitoring	Monitoring intervals, data to be monitored, scales to be used.
Response evaluation criteria or endpoints	Traditional endpoints in determining the toxicity of a new drug are survival rate, disease-free survival rate, response rate, duration of response and treatment toxicity. The major endpoint of phase I trials is toxicity. Evaluation of any tumour response is a secondary endpoint. Endpoints of phase II and III trials may vary.
Statistical considerations	Statistical analyses to be performed.
Criteria for study termination	Situations that require cessation of the study.

■ **BOX 6.2** *(Continued)*

Special companion studies	Studies complementary or parallel to the clinical study.
References	References relevant for the study rationale and interpretation of results.
Consent form	The informed consent form to be signed by the patient.

Adapted from Melink & Whitacre (1991).

■ **BOX 6.3   Good Clinical Practices**

Good Clinical Practices (GCPs) originated from the 1976 Congressional recommendations of the US Food and Drug Administration. They consist of a set of rules that govern clinical investigations, in order to protect patients' rights and also to guarantee the methodologically correct conduct of a clinical trial. GCPs involve the procedural aspects of conducting and monitoring a clinical trial, and specifically:

- responsibility of the investigators.
- responsibilities of the sponsor.
- requirements for approval of the trial.
- requirements for monitoring data collection in different centres. This includes site visits to verify compliance with regulatory issues, protocol specifications and data accuracy; this is generally obtained by comparing the original patient record with the data collected in the research form.
- standards for obtaining informed consent.

supportive therapies, psychological interventions and biological agents. Trials may also evaluate the effectiveness of programmes of cancer prevention and control, the psychological impact of the illness and treatments on patients, and the effectiveness of diagnostic tests and programmes.

Different types of clinical trial

To develop a new anticancer drug, and use it in human beings, there are several steps to be followed and different kind of studies to be implemented. The main stages and characteristics of each step are outlined below.

Phase I studies

The aim of phase I studies is to determine toxicities and the optimal or maximum tolerated dose (MTD), and to investigate the pharmacokinetics of the agent. These studies are conducted in subjects with advanced cancer, for which no other effective therapy exists. In phase I cancer clinical trials it is necessary to involve patients with cancer (rather than healthy volunteers), owing to the potentially toxic nature of the drugs. The disease itself and drug interactions may change the metabolism of the drug (Holdener, Decoster & Lim 1992).

In phase I studies, pharmacological data on drug absorption, distribution and metabolism are also needed, requiring frequent urine and blood sample collection in some patients. Pharmacological evaluations are conducted with each schedule variation in order to determine the beneficial and adverse effects of dose and schedule. A phase I study is generally considered complete when a MTD is identified, even in the absence of objective antitumour response. The lack of antitumour activity in this phase is not evidence for the ineffectiveness of the drug. An agent with antitumour activity may not produce objective and/or significant antitumour effect during the early phases of a study. This may be a consequence of the fact that the optimal dosage and schedule of administration is not yet known (as well as the toxic side-effects on human tissue). Traditionally, the initial dose administered is one-tenth of the MTD in mice during clinical toxicology studies. Less than 4% of the patients entering phase I trials will achieve an objective response (i.e. not biased by the doctor's personal opinion), but they have a high chance of experiencing unwanted side-effects (Estey et al 1986).

Phase II studies

The aim of phase II studies is to determine the effectiveness of an agent in one or more types of cancer. Patients enrolled in the study must have measurable disease and a life expectancy long enough to permit observation of the drug effect. New-generation phase II studies are disease specific: the choice of the disease is based on the data collected during a phase I study and/or *in vitro* test results. In designing phase II studies, variables such as pretreatment with chemotherapy, performance status and extent of the disease must be considered, and study objectives must be clearly defined. Additional pharmacological data collected during phase II studies improve knowledge of the drug (Jenkins & Hubbard 1991). Such studies must accrue a sufficient number of patients in order to obtain statistically meaningful conclusions.

Phase III studies

Phase III studies aim to define the role of a new treatment (drug, drug combination, procedure, etc.) in the management of the patient in terms of survival and quality of life. In other words, phase III studies compare the agent with other treatments to demonstrate whether the agent or regimen is more effective than the standard therapy (or as effective, but associated with less morbidity). A phase III trial is conducted only if the new treatment is equivalent or better as compared to the standard therapy. Phase III trials are generally controlled studies (with an experimental and control group); they are randomized (i.e. subjects are assigned to treatments by chance); outcomes are established by statistical analysis; and an adequate number of patients must be recruited. Generally these studies require the participation of several institutions following the same protocol (collaborative or multicentre studies). The expected differences in order to document the advantages of the new treatment must be identified and stated in advance. These trials may be double-blind (i.e. neither the patient nor the investigator knows which treatment is administered). A phase III trial can be stopped before its completion if the evidence so far produced is significantly better in favour of one treatment compared with another (Jenkins & Hubbard 1991).

Phase IV studies

Phase IV studies involve the use of a new therapy in practice, but with systematic monitoring and recording of outcome data.

Nurses' involvement in medical clinical trials

In the past, a nurse's role was mainly identified as that of medical–clinical data collector. Nurses are now considered an essential component of the clinical trials research process. Collaboration between doctors and nurses and an experienced multidisciplinary team is, in fact, pivotal to the initiation and conduct of a trial. Nurses' role in clinical trials was explored in a survey that involved 120 nurses (38% of the nurses originally contacted) from 15 different countries across Europe (Arrigo et al 1994). The list of tasks and activities mainly performed by nurses when they participate in the organization and management of medical clinical trials is illustrated in Table 6.3.

Nurses may undertake a number of different roles and their involvement may vary from standard tasks related to patient care and data collection for the trial, to full involvement in the design and implementation of the research project and the interpretation of the results. Suggestions from nurses as to how to improve their participation in clinical trials include: courses (73%), seminars (68%), practical training (60%), symposia (51%), newsletters (44%) and brochures (36%) (Arrigo et al 1994). Basic requirements for nurses to participate in a clinical trial include having a clear understanding of the study protocol and making sure it is also understood by the other staff members. The protocol should ideally be presented and discussed before initiation of the study, and aspects relevant to nursing care should be discussed. As is evident from Table 6.3, nurses can have an instrumental and independent role in clinical trials.

Nurses' role in clinical trials

Nurses have the potential to perform a broader role than that identified by Arrigo and colleagues (1994). Nurses' participation in clinical trials is, in fact, very stimulating and challenging. It requires a large compendium of skills, which research nurses and staff nurses have developed in a complementary fashion (Cassidy & McFarlane

Table 6.3 Results of the EORTC–ONSG (European Organization for Research and Treatment of Cancer–Oncology Nurses Study Group) survey on nurses' tasks and activities in clinical trials

	Yes respondents (%)
Tasks	
Patient information	74
Drug administration	65
Monitoring of toxicities	62
Organization of follow-up	55
Basic patient care	50
Data management	50
Drug preparation	46
Activities	
Supplying information to nursing colleagues	77
Participation in patient information	73
Participation in obtaining informed consent	56
Writing of nursing summaries	48
Participation in writing protocols	29
Participation in protocol scientific review	21
Participation in ethical review	13

Adapted from Arrigo et al (1994).

1991, McEvoy, Cannon & McDermott 1991). The research nurse, where available, is responsible for coordinating nursing care in order that the patient included in the research protocol receives optimal care. She also plays the role of coordinator, educator, patient ally and, sometimes, direct caregiver. The staff nurse can also perform all of these roles when the research nurse is not available.

Different roles of a nurse in cancer clinical trials

Direct caregiver Direct caregiving is, and remains, the core activity of most nurses; according to Arrigo et al (1994), this comprises 65% of all the activities performed by nurses involved in clinical trials. Patients involved in clinical trials do continue to need basic nursing care, together with psychological support and closer observation. Nurses need to answer to patients' needs but also to identify potential side-effects and toxicities of treatment. The planning of the complex nursing care required helps to prevent problems and ensures patient safety. Maintaining the continuity of care significantly contributes to the physical and emotional well-being of patients included in research protocols.

Administration of investigative therapy The research nurse and staff nurse (when a research nurse is not available) are responsible for the delivery of treatments to be administered, according to the research protocol (McEvoy, Cannon & McDermott 1991). Very often, the treatment regimens include complex drug administration patterns, frequent blood sampling, and close patient observation and monitoring. When pharmacokinetic questions are asked in addition to those that relate to toxicity, the times at which blood samples are drawn and the amount of fluid provided to the patient may be critical.

Observation of treatment-related side-effects The nurse is responsible for the observation and early recognition of side-effects of treatments in general (Wheeler 1991). Nurses should also be aware of the criteria for assessing the response to a therapy and for terminating the protocol. The patient must be taught, and often reminded, to report any known or suspected toxicities or any unusual or unexpected symptoms.

Patient advocacy The nurse adopts responsibility for patient information. Even when not closely involved in the research protocol, the nurse has the responsibility of assessing how much the patient is informed and aware of the situation, and how much he or she understands any information provided (Meili 1991). Patient and family information is the cornerstone of any patient's decision to participate in a clinical trial. The nurse has the responsibility of supporting patients in the informed consent procedure, of helping them to clarify the reasons for participating in the clinical trial and/or withdrawing from treatment when the patient desires it.

Informing the patient in an adequate manner requires experience and skills. In fact, because of the stressful nature of the experience (coupled, for some patients, with social and cultural factors), the patient may not be receptive to any information provided. Information to be shared with the patient mainly includes what might be experienced while undergoing the treatment and information on the treatment itself – where it will be delivered, frequency of delivery, who will administer it, side-effects likely to be experienced and monitoring procedures.

Organization of the study Nurses can create an atmosphere that motivates protocol patients to return for therapy and tests at specified times (Cassidy & McFarlane 1991). This can also include the preparation of specific written materials for the patient. It is generally accepted that a greater understanding of any situation enhances or improves cooperation. Patient motivation and a clear explanation of their role and responsibilities are also of the utmost importance. The extra burden of work related to the clinical trials activities is sometimes not compatible with the everyday caring activities, so clinical research units have been created (Cameron 1997). Such units have been specifically established for patients undergoing phase I clinical trials, since these are the most intensive, particularly in terms of nursing care and support.

Staff educator When the nurse holds the position of coordinator she is responsible for setting up communication and decision-making strategies (Crawford et al 1990). Nurses involved in clinical trials (especially research nurses) should inform or educate other colleagues on the principles of clinical trials and the contents of the research protocol, in order to improve patient observation and care.

Role of the nurse in informed consent

Once the patient is deemed eligible for entry to a protocol, the procedures related to the obtaining informed consent should be followed. The main ethical issues encountered during the conduct of phase I studies have recently been summarized:

- Treatment of patients at ineffective or toxic doses
- Low probability of response
- Unknown toxic effects and benefits of the new agent
- Difficulty of obtaining adequate informed consent in vulnerable patients
- Lack of accord between the objectives of the investigators and those of the patients.

Informed consent is a necessary requirement for the patient's involvement in any kind of research. A member of the medical staff should be available to answer any questions and, after receipt of information, the patient (or legally authorized representative) is generally asked to sign the informed consent form. Only after this step can the patient be randomized or registered on a protocol. In the past, the role of the nurse in the informed consent procedure was limited to verification that the signature on the form was that of the patient and of witnessing that the patient had signed the form; the changing role of the nurse and the autonomy of the expanded roles brings new professional and ethical responsibilities (Meili 1991). More and more often, nurses are involved in explaining the details of the protocol and the consent form and in the assessment of a patient's ability to understand verbal and written instructions and information.

An informed consent process, as the words imply, is neither a task nor a formal ritual limited to a signature on a form, but rather it is a process of shared decision-making based on participation and mutual respect. Even when a patient has given consent to entering a trial, the nurse should continually assess their integration of new knowledge and understanding of the research treatment (Meili 1991). Consent to participate in research is valid only if voluntary (i.e. free from coercion and from the influences of other persons). In reality, we are rarely entirely free of various pressures, and a fully voluntary choice is clearly an ideal (Grady 1991). If and how much the consent is really informed is still the object of debate (Fallowfield et al 1998, Tognoni & Geraci 1997).

Very often, nurses and doctors are worried that the informed consent could affect the doctor–nurse–patient relationship. Patients receiving detailed information have a better understanding of investigational therapies and procedures, a decreased willingness to participate in randomization, but no significant difference in their perception of the physician–patient relationship (Simes et al 1986). No recommended procedure exists for the collection of informed consent. An atmosphere of open communication, trust and warmth are essential ingredients. The patient should be given the opportunity to think over the information given, ask for further explanations and discuss it with relatives, as necessary. Nurses can be of great emotional and informational support in this process and very often are the professionals from whom the patient asks for further information and clarification. Ways of assessing the adequateness of the informed consent procedure and the patient's level of understanding have been proposed (Tomamichel et al 1995).

Role of the nurse in quality-of-life data collection

Quality of life (QoL) is increasingly being used as a complementary endpoint to the traditional outcomes of mortality and morbidity to evaluate the impact of new treatments on patients with cancer, recognizing that it is not cure and survival alone that are important (Editorial 1995). Three times as many articles were published on this subject in 1994 as in 1990, and QoL is being recognized as a major endpoint for phase III randomized controlled trials (Editorial 1991).

The concept of QoL (or even health-related QoL) extends far beyond health status, encompassing many other areas and activities of life such as the psychological domain, level of independence, social relationships, environment, spirituality, religion and personal beliefs (World Health Organization Quality of Life Group 1995). The importance of good health in achieving a high perceived QoL lies in the extent to which it enhances, limits or prevents the enjoyment of work, family life, leisure and other activities (Ruta et al 1994).

Measurement of QoL is important to identify vulnerable periods in the patient's health–illness continuum, in order to provide more support and to anticipate times when QoL is at a low point. It may enable nurses to evaluate the impact of medical and nursing interventions on patients' lives in terms of things that matter to them most.

We know that a patient's self-assessment may differ substantially from the judgement of a doctor or other healthcare professionals (Sprangers & Aaronson 1992). Many patients accept toxic chemotherapy for the prospect of a slight benefit, contrary to the expectations of healthcare professionals; therefore QoL should be self-assessed by the patient. Although in the literature there is a raging debate on QoL measurements (Corner 1997, Gill & Fenstein 1994, Leplege & Hunt 1997), nurses are often asked and made responsible for the collection of QoL data in clinical trials.

QoL data collection requires a reasonable amount of planning. Assessment times should be planned according to patient visits. Although questionnaires are designed to be self-administered, patients need explanation, support and motivation in order to spend the time completing them (the amount of time required to complete a QoL questionnaire may range from a few minutes to more than half an hour, and may further vary according to the patient's health conditions). Therefore, questionnaire administration should be planned according to nursing workload and nurses should be informed of the aims of the QoL study.

Nursing summaries

In spite of the long-term participation of nurses in clinical trials, suggestions as to how to improve or increase their participation are rare in the literature. The high workload of oncology units often leaves nurses with little time to read the entire protocol document (Meili 1991). Very often, clinical trial protocols do not provide detailed practical instructions on the delivery of the treatments, the observation and documentation of their effects on patients, and the management of complications. Strict adherence to the protocol is a particularly important requirement, especially for multicentre studies, to counter different monitoring policies or variation in medical and nursing practices. In fact, variations in the management of side-effects or in supportive care, and the ranges and intervals of monitoring, may lead to delay in the identification of complications and in the decision to stop the research treatment.

■ **BOX 6.4   Possible list of contents for a nursing summary**

Name of protocol

Responsible investigator

Phase I, II or III study

Aims of the study

Patient population

Patient selection criteria (relevant to nurses)

Protocol design/treatment regimens

Drug information:

- stability
- solution in which it is diluted
- how long it is stable once mixed
- how to be administered.

Potential side-effects, toxicity, nursing problems, diagnoses

Nursing interventions required

Points of special attention

Pharmacokinetic studies:

- list of blood samples
- how the blood is to be collected
- what will be done with the sample (centrifuging, storage).

   Lab requirements

   Evaluation of toxicity

   Follow-up procedure

Modified from Di Giulio et al (1996).

Nursing summaries of clinical research protocols provide nurses with a short and easy-to-read selection of relevant information about the study. It should supply shorthand information on the more practical aspects of the research protocol and thus render easier, time-saving and safer the implementation of the research protocol (Di Giulio et al 1996). Nursing summaries should not be considered easy and simplified summaries of the research protocol, but complementary research protocols that stress aspects of patient daily treatment and observation. The basic structure and contents of a nursing summary are proposed in Box 6.4. The nursing summary can be prepared by the protocol team; it can identify significant questions and information left unanswered or not dealt with sufficiently in the main protocol, and suggest practical solutions. The variability of nursing roles and caring environments will require customization of the nursing summary to local needs. The level of detail to be provided in a nursing summary should be discussed locally in order to render the nursing summary a helpful instrument in different local situations.

Companion studies

Nurses' roles in clinical trials are not limited to collaboration with doctors. Nurses can organize independent trials or studies associated with a clinical trial.

Table 6.4 Benefits and barriers involved in conducting companion studies

Benefits	Barriers
Enhanced access to subjects	A companion study needs to be designed as independent study, although compatible with other counterparts
Opportunity for independent research	Often viewed as second-class studies
Efficiency in data collection	Subject burden may be increased with multiple outcome measures
More comprehensive appraisal of patient outcomes	Analysis of study results, ownership of data, and plans for dissemination through publication or presentation need to be negotiated in advance
Opportunity for multicentre research	Collaboration and communication between investigators is time consuming
Cost and organizational burden containment	Compatibility of protocols is necessary to avoid conflicting methods

Modified from Ferrel & Cohen (1991).

Collaborative companion studies are those studies associated with an existing medical study, which may involve interdisciplinary effort of both nurse and physicians. The two protocols are conducted jointly and there is a significant overlap in subject accrual, data collection and the day-to-day management of the study. Companion studies may also parallel a clinical trial, initiated in response to a (nursing) concern that may have been generated by the observation of patients in an ongoing medical study (Ferrel & Cohen 1991).

In some countries, nurses have little opportunity to recruit patients for nurse-led studies, or to ask patients to come back to the hospital or clinic in order to fill out questionnaires or to have a nursing assessment. Companion studies represent the opportunity to promote easier access to patients, to improve subject accrual and to share the organizational burden and costs. Moreover, they offer the opportunity for interdisciplinary work. Table 6.4 summarizes the benefits and barriers in conducting companion studies. The main topics that nursing companion studies have focused upon include treatment effects or symptoms such as pain, nutritional concerns, mucositis, nausea and QoL (Ferrel & Cohen 1991). Other common areas are cancer control and rehabilitation.

How to prepare nurses for clinical trials

Many authors agree that clinical nurses are a vital component in the success and implementation of a clinical trial (Wheeler 1991). In some cases, nurses' participation in clinical trials is rendered very difficult by the lack of clarity associated with their role, by the high workload, the conflict of responsibilities, the lack of nursing education in research methodology, and the poor recognition generally awarded to nurses involved in research activities (Johansen, Mayer & Hoover 1991).

One of the important responsibilities of the educator in preparing staff for the initiation of a new protocol is to analyse the impact of the study on nurses and nursing care. Questions important for such evaluation involve an assessment of toxicities, the time required for assessing the patient, for administering treatments, and for the monitoring of the patient (laboratory examinations, specific storage or handling requirements). A clear knowledge of the incidence and severity of side-effects in order to plan the intensity of nursing care required to balance patient needs is required, for example the intensity of emesis and the need for cardiac monitoring (Wheeler 1991). Several areas require further planning, for example:

1. If unfamiliar equipment has to be implemented for drug administration, then time for instruction and training should be planned for in order to facilitate the acquisition of the necessary skills to administer treatment safely.

2. The implementation of a new protocol may result in admission to the ward of patients with whom nurses are unfamiliar, for example extremely severely ill patients or those with kidney or lung problems. Staff nurses may not be familiar with assessment, recognition and treatment of these conditions. Basic knowledge on how to handle the most common patient problems should be provided before initiation of the trial.

3. The opportunity of developing specific information materials should be considered when planning time and resources needed for the study. This kind of assessment can be conducted in the planning phase by the project group, or by the nursing group, before the start of the protocol.

The roles and activities described are important not only to guarantee the patients' safety but also to protect nurses' rights. Besides participating in the clinical trial, the primary nurse must continue to deliver patient care; if nurses are not provided with the right information and support, this often hampers initial enthusiasm and nurses are left with anger and frustration that leads to the possibility of them being unsupportive of future clinical research (Johansen, Mayer & Hoover 1991).

RESEARCH RESOURCE DEVELOPMENT IN EUROPE

Adequate support for cancer nursing research is a critical factor in realizing our research agenda. Support from nursing colleagues both within and outwith the specialty, and from members of other healthcare disciplines such as medicine, is critical to initiating a successful research proposal (Grant 1990). The need for financial support varies, depending on the nature of the study. Some research can be carried out with little or no financial support. However, financial support is often crucial to the successful implementation of both data collection and analysis, especially when a project involves a substantial number of collaborators and multiple sites. The need for significant financial support will become increasingly more likely as cancer nurse researchers in Europe seek to design and implement studies that will have a greater degree of generalizability across Europe.

Unfortunately, financial support for cancer nursing research in Europe is limited. Whilst, as has been noted above, some research can be carried out with just a minimum level of resources, most projects require some level of support for the key activities of data collection, data management and analysis, and project management. Some sponsors may require applications that have a collaborative element, and the process of trying to secure funding for such a project can involve a great deal of time and energy in the preparation and submission of a proposal, but such projects also hold significant elements. Additional income generated through the funding of such a project can enhance the scope of the research, whilst also facilitating the forging of effective relations both with the collaborators and the organization that has funded the study.

Submitting a research proposal for funding

The receipt of early information on potential research opportunities is a prerequisite for a successful proposal. Bond's (1994) comment that 'many research projects never see the light of day because researchers fail to get the grant application right' (p. 34) is one that should be well heeded by prospective researchers. Too many potentially good proposals are rejected because applicants did not allow themselves sufficient time to prepare and present proposals that met the criteria of a prospective project sponsor. Some organizations have pre-set dates each year for the receipt of applications, whilst others issue periodic calls for proposals. Such a distinction is important to understand. In cases of the initiated mode (i.e. a submission to a call for proposals from a body wishing to provide funding for a specific topic), there is often a willingness only to fund research in line with pre-defined topics and to a defined budget. This often constitutes the approach adopted by governmental bodies or national nursing organizations, which expect individual researchers or teams to submit an application in line with a tight specification. Alternatively, a grant application is initiated by the researcher themselves, and the awarding body responds – an approach consistent with many of the major medical and nursing charities and foundations. Whichever method is pursued, it is vital to keep abreast of the range and timing of opportunities that are available. The first source of information should be one's own institution, but in addition to this there are several publications that detail research funding and training opportunities.

Most research sponsors provide some level of detail on the subject area for which they are interested in receiving proposals. Naturally, proposals should always address these identified topics or subject areas (see Box 6.5 for guidance on submitting an application for funding). It is not always helpful to suggest alternative means of achieving research objectives when the funder clearly advises the nature of their priorities in their call for proposals. As most proposals are submitted to some level of peer group review, and as the programmes themselves may be extremely competitive, it is important that answers are provided to the questions that are asked, and not the question that might have been posed.

Most proposals are assessed on their scientific quality, originality and compliance with the aims of the programme in question. However, when submitting a proposal, it may be useful to consider the following questions:

- What are the objectives of the research, and what method will be used to meet these objectives?
- What are the advantages and benefits that will arise as a result of the study?
- What are the anticipated milestones in connection with the project plan?
- Are the costs required to complete the project eligible under the terms of the programme?
- Why is the applicant(s) and their proposed study particularly suited to meeting the desired aims of the research programme?
- Are there any particular ethical considerations and constraints?
- Does the applicant(s) have sufficient expertise to complete the proposed study, or are partners desirable or required?

■ BOX 6.5 Six steps to ensure the success of a research proposal submitted for funding

---

- Early receipt of information on funding opportunities.
- Fully address the requirements of the funding organization.
- Provide accurate and realistic costings.
- Involve effective collaborators when warranted.
- Make good use of professional help.
- Timely submission of the finished proposal.

Explicit guidance about the form to be taken by proposals is often offered and should be followed to the letter. Many sponsors now require that applications are submitted on pre-designed forms (often issued on disk) and in multiple copies. Proposals should be fully and accurately costed, bearing in mind that costs may have to be justified at the time of the contract negotiation and most funders will not allow any additional amounts to be added to your budget (e.g. if no provision for salary increases was included in the costings that were submitted). It is always useful to seek assistance from a financial officer familiar with costing research proposals. Many universities have departments dedicated to the support of research, which includes assisting with the formulation of a quality application and the ongoing administration of a research grant. If this is not available, most funding bodies are willing to provide additional guidance. Costs are normally classified under two headings: direct and indirect.

Direct costs are costs that are directly attributable to the project, such as labour costs, travel and subsistence, consumables, equipment, data management costs, publications, specific communications costs (e.g. telephone and fax) and any sub-contracts.

Indirect costs (also known as overheads) are usually used by an organization to maintain the infrastructure that is necessary to support research activities and may include: personnel administration, financial support, salary administration, legal services, cleaning costs, building maintenance, library services, etc. The application form and supporting documentation will normally detail those costs that are deemed 'allowable' or 'eligible', but it is wise to seek further clarification over any items of expenditure for which there is a degree of ambiguity.

Sources of help and advice

For help and advice, the first point of contact should be your local institution. Most universities and colleges, for example, have research support offices that can offer a wide range of services to applicants, including helping to identify possible sources of funding, the preparation and costing of applications, and the negotiation of contracts. If more specialist information and/or advice is required, then most funding bodies have staff who act as programme contact points and who will provide further assistance to prospective applicants.

The European Commission (EC) is an example of an organization that has a strong support network, with most programmes having delegated officials for each research area. If you intend to apply to the EC for research funding, you may also wish to contact your local EuroInfoCentre (EIC) for information and advice. The network of EICs was established by the EC in 1987 and comprises around 230 centres in the member states of the European Union plus Norway and Iceland.

Research funding opportunities

Funding for research is available from a variety of sources. One of the first, and most logical, sources to pursue for financial support is one's own institution. This is especially appropriate if the investigator has limited or no grant-writing experience (Grant 1990). In educational institutions, funds are sometimes available that are intended to promote research amongst the faculty, or through the result of a bequest, often given with the intention of supporting a scholarship or funding postgraduate studies in a defined area of interest. In clinical settings, financial support may be available through the provision of bursaries or scholarships, which are won through a competitive process, and often coordinated by the continuing education or quality assurance department. The amount of funds made available through such a route may be smaller than that from charitable or governmental sources;

however, it is an excellent source for small pilot studies, and can of course be combined with several other small awards in order to conduct a more substantial project.

Local, national and international charities, private foundations and grant-making trusts are also often a useful source of support for funding applications. Their funding priorities tend to be well defined and the application process may be reasonably straightforward, sometimes with a relatively quick decision being made on a successful application.

Inhabitants of individual countries will be able to access government funds available to support research and practice development, which may be obtained through city, regional or national/federal sources. Publications are often available that list grant programmes and deadline dates. Funding may be available either to support a project where the idea has been developed into a proposal by the investigator or, alternatively, to support the conduct of a particular piece of research, where the idea and focus of the study have been developed by the funding agency. Obviously, commercial and industrial sources, principally pharmaceutical companies, will remain a valuable source of funding.

The EC is a major provider of funding for collaborative research in Europe, although for most programmes there must be effective collaboration between at least two investigators in at least two of the 15 Member States. The proposals must be innovative and the results of the project capable of exploitation or commercialization. The Commission funds research via a multiannual Framework Programme which comprises a number of individual research programmes, covering a range of scientific areas. The Fourth Framework Programme ran from 1994 to 1998 and comprised 15 individual research programmes plus other activities dealing with cooperation with non-EC countries, dissemination and training and mobility of researchers. The latter made fellowships available to enable young scientists to undertake PhDs or to fund postdoctoral research, tenable in a different member state to that of the nationality of the applicant. The Fifth Framework Programme (FPV) runs from 1998 to 2002, with a total budget of 14 960 million Euros. The 'Quality of Life and Management of Living Resources' and the 'Improving Human Potential' programmes are of particular interest to cancer nurses. Full details of FPV, including the individual research areas covered by these programmes, can be found on the Commission's website http://www.cordis.lu/fp5/home.html, or may be sought in writing from the following address: European Commission, DGXII.E.8., Square de Meeus, B-1040 Brussels, Belgium. Applications to the EC can involve a great deal of time and effort, and it is wise to seek expert assistance from a local support office.

At present, cancer nursing research is generally disadvantaged in competing successfully for research funds, largely due to insufficient interest and inadequate infrastructure to enable competitive applications to be submitted. Cancer nursing research must be able to compete on equal terms with medical research projects. The prime need is to generate bids of high quality that will enable nursing projects to gain access to the research agendas of funding bodies, and therefore compete on equal terms with other projects, and where necessary to encourage greater willingness among these bodies to examine cancer nursing proposal on their merits.

CONCLUSION

The development and maintenance of nursing research in Europe has been recognized as a priority, 'enabling professional practice to be rationalised and assessed, thus helping to improve the quality of individual and community care, whether preventive, curative, palliative or aimed at integration' (European Health Committee 1996, p. 1). Meeting the research needs of nurses in cancer care will remain a challenge as we enter the next century. Nurses will have to continue to acquire and increase the means necessary to enable the informed critique, conduct and, where warranted, implementation of research. In order to base cancer nursing practice on evidence, the evidence has – to put it bluntly – first to be generated and, second, evaluated. Cancer nurses need to demand and obtain the resources, whether they be in terms of human resources, material or money (Arrigo 1991), to ensure that the conduct of these two activities are continually strengthened. European cancer nurses need to continue to mature in confidence when it comes to researching their own practice and developing the science and art of cancer nursing. Likewise, it is vital to foster the confidence of others so that research work can attract funding.

Research in the field is gaining momentum. Hopes of increasing the productivity of individual studies may well depend on the extent to which we are willing to enter into collaborative efforts with others, within and outwith our profession. Collaborative studies, by involving a number of investigators in several settings, can solve many problems and difficulties, most notably that of sample size. They are also useful for testing from the outset the effectiveness of interventions in multiple settings and with personnel of varying skills and abilities (Oberst 1979), so often the case in Europe. Serious exploration of the potential of European research groups to address some of the major research questions facing cancer nursing must be executed post-haste.

REFERENCES

Arrigo C 1991 Meeting the research needs of nurses in cancer care. European Journal of Cancer Care 1(1):19–22

Arrigo C, Gall H, Delogne A, Molin C 1994 The involvement of nurses in clinical trials. Results of the EORTC Oncology Nurses Study Group review. Cancer Nursing 17(5): 429–433.

Bond S 1994 Writing a grant application. Nurse Researcher 2(1):31–35

Cameron C 1997 The clinical research unit: a nurse led unit for patients undergoing early anti-cancer drug trials. Journal of Cancer Nursing 1(1):32–36

Cassidy J, McFarlane D 1991 The role of the nurse in clinical cancer research. Cancer Nursing 14(3):124–131

Cawley N, Webber J 1995 Research priorities in palliative care. International Journal of Palliative Nursing 1(2):101–113

Corner J 1991 Cancer nursing in Europe: beyond 2000. European Journal of Cancer Care 1(1):11–14

Corner J 1993 Building a framework for nursing research in cancer care. European Journal of Cancer Care 2(3):112–116

Corner J 1997 Beyond survival rates and side effects: cancer nursing as therapy. Cancer Nursing 20(1):3–11.

Crane J 1995 The future of research utilisation. Nursing Clinics of North America 30:565–577.

Crawford S, Beardsley R, Lamy P, Mech A, Proksch R 1990 Comparing fact sheets and lectures to provide investigational drug information. Journal of Nursing and Staff Development 6(1):35–39

Degner L 1984 The status of cancer nursing research in Canada. Nursing Papers 16:4–13

Denton S 1996 Exploring the impact of treatment: communications, perceptions, reality! European Journal of Cancer Care 5(suppl 3):3–4

Di Giulio P, Arrigo C, Gall H, Molin C, Nieweg R, Strohbucker B 1996 Expanding the role of the nurse in clinical trials: nursing summaries. Cancer Nursing 19(5):343–347

Editorial 1991 Quality of life. Lancet 338:350–351

Editorial 1995 Quality of life and clinical trials. Lancet 346:1–2

Estey E, Hoth H, Simon R, Marsoni S, Leyland-Jones B, Wites R 1986 Therapeutic response in phase 1 trials of antineoplastic agents. Cancer Treatment Reports 70(1):71–80

European Health Committee (1996) Nursing research – report and recommendations. Council of Europe, Strasburg

European Oncology Nursing Society 1992 A core curriculum on research for nurses in cancer care. EONS, Brussels

Fallowfield L, Jenkins V, Brennan C, Sawtell M, Moynihan C, Souhami R 1998 Attitudes of patients to randomised clinical trials of cancer therapy. European Journal of Cancer 34:1554–1559

Fernsler J, Holcombe J, Pulliam L 1984 A survey of cancer nursing research. Oncology Nursing Forum 11(4):46–52

Ferrel B, Cohen M 1991 Companion studies. Seminars in Oncology Nursing 7(4):252–259

Fitch M 1996 ISNCC launches research initiative. International Cancer Nursing News 8(3):13

Fitch M, Thompson L 1996 Fostering the growth of research-based oncology nursing practice. Oncology Nursing Forum 23(4):631–637

Funk S, Champagne M, Wiese R, Tornquist E 1991 BARRIERS: the barriers to research utilization scale. Applied Nursing Research 4(1):90–95

Funk S, Tonquist E, Champagne M 1995 Barriers and facilitators of research utilisation: an integrative review. Nursing Clinics of North America 30:395–407

Funkhouser S, Grant M 1989 1988 ONS survey of research priorities. Oncology Nursing Forum 16:413–416

Gill T, Fenstein A 1994 A critical appraisal of quality of life measurements. Journal of the American Medical Association 272(8):619–626

Grady C 1991 Ethical issues in clinical trials. Seminars in Oncology Nursing 7(4):288–296

Grant M 1990 Support for research. In: Grant M, Padilla G (eds) Cancer nursing research: a practical approach. Appleton & Lange, Norwalk, Connecticut, p 163

Grant M, Padilla G 1983 An overview of cancer nursing research. Oncology Nursing Forum 10(1):58–67

Grant M, Stromborg M 1981 Promoting research collaboration: ONS Research Committee survey. Oncology Nursing Forum 8(2):48–53

Graydon J, West P, Galloway S et al 1993 Bridging the gap between research and clinical practice: a collaborative approach. Oncology Nursing Forum 20(6):953–957

Holdener E, Decoster G, Lim C 1992 Ethical aspects of phase 1 studies in cancer patients. In: Willimans C (ed) Introducing new treatments for cancer: practical, ethical and legal problems. John Wiley, Chichester, UK, p 157

Hopwood P 1996 A checklist for patients on endocrine therapy (C-PET). European Journal of Cancer Care 5(suppl 3):7–8

Jenkins J, Hubbard S 1991 History of clinical trials. Seminars in Oncology Nursing 7(4):228–234

Jodrell N 1996 Workflow Information Systems for European Nursing Care (WISECARE). University of Edinburgh, Edinburgh

Johansen M, Mayer D, Hoover H 1991 Obstacles to implementing cancer clinical trials. Seminars In Oncology Nursing 7(4):260–267

Leplege A, Hunt S 1997 The problem of quality of life in medicine. Journal of the American Medical Association 278(1):47–50

McCorkle R, Lewis F 1980 Research in cancer nursing. Seminars in Oncology Nursing 7(1):80–87

McEvoy M, Cannon L, McDermott M 1991 The professional role of the nurse in clinical trials. Seminars in Oncology Nursing 7(4):268–274

McGuire D, Harwood K 1989 The CNS as researcher. In: Hamric A, Spross J (eds) The clinical nurse specialist in theory and practice. W B Saunders, Philadelphia, p 169

McGuire D, Frank-Stromborg M, Varricchio C 1985 1984 ONS Research Committee survey of membership's research interests and involvement. Oncology Nursing Forum 12(2):99–103

McGuire D, Walczak J, Krumm S 1994 Development of a nursing research utilization programme in a clinical oncology setting: organisation, implementation, and evaluation. Oncology Nursing Forum 21(4):704–710

Meili L 1991 The community hospital perspective of clinical trials and the role of the nurse educator. Seminars in Oncology Nursing 7(4):280–287

Melink T, Whitacre Y 1991 Planning and implementing clinical trials. Seminars in Oncology Nursing 7(4):243–251

Mooney K, Haberman M 1996 Cancer nursing research today. In: McCorkle R, Grant M, Frank-Stromborg M, Baird S (eds) Cancer nursing. A comprehensive textbook. W B Saunders, Philadelphia, p 1261

Mooney K, Ferrell B, Nail L, Benedict S, Haberman M 1991 1991 Oncology Nursing Society research priorities survey. Oncology Nursing Forum 18:1381–1388

Nieweg R, Ambaum B, Teunissen S et al 1996 Research priorities in oncology nursing in the Netherlands (abstract no. 345). In: ISNCC (ed) Ninth international conference on cancer nursing, 12–15 August 1996. RCN Publishing Brighton, UK

Oberst M 1978 Priorities in cancer nursing research. Cancer Nursing 1:281–290

Oberst M 1979 Problems and potential in cancer nursing research. Cancer Nursing 2(4), 305–306

Padilla G 1990 Progress in cancer nursing research. In: Grant M, Padilla G (eds) Cancer nursing research: a practical approach. Appleton & Lange, Norwalk, Connecticut, p 9

Payne S 1993 Constraints for nursing in developing a framework for cancer care research. European Journal of Cancer Care 2(3):117–120

Richardson A, Wilson-Barnet J 1995 A review of nursing research in cancer and palliative care. In: Richardson A, Wilson-Barnett J (eds) Nursing research in cancer care. Scutari Press, London, p 1

Ruta D, Garrat, A, Leng M, Russel I, McDonald L 1994 A new approach to the measurement of quality of life. The patient generated index. Medical Care 32(11):1109–1126.

Rutledge D, Ropka M, Greene P, Nail L, Mooney K 1998 Barriers to research utilisation for oncology staff nurses and nurse manager/clinical nurse specialists. Oncology Nursing Forum, 25(3):497–506

Simes R, Tattershall M, Coates A et al 1986 Randomised comparison of procedures for obtaining informed consent in clinical trials of treatment for cancer. British Medical Journal 293:1065–1068

Smith M, Stullenberger E 1995 An integrative review and meta-analysis of oncology nursing research: 1981–1991. Cancer Nursing 18(3):167–179

Smith M, Holcombe J, Stullenberger E 1994 A meta-analysis of intervention effectiveness for symptom management in oncology nursing research. Oncology Nursing Forum 21, 1201–1209

Sprangers M, Aaronson N 1992 The role of health care providers and significant others in evaluating the quality of life of patients with chronic disease: a review. Journal of Clinical Epidemiology 45(7):743–760

Stetler C 1994 Refinement of the Stetler/Marram model for application of research findings to practice. Nursing Outlook 42:15–25

Stetz K, Haberman M, Holcombe J, Jones L 1995 1994 Oncology Nursing Society research priorities survey. Oncology Nursing Forum 22(5):785–789

Stone K 1991 Collaboration. In: Mateo M, Kirchoff K (eds) Conducting and using research in the clinical setting. Williams & Wilkins, Baltimore, p 58

Tierney A 1994 The development of nursing research in Europe: keynote paper. In: Seventh Workshop of European Nurse Researchers (WENR). WENR, Oslo

Tierney A 1997 The development of nursing research in Europe. European Nurse 2(2): 73–84

Tognoni, G, Geraci E 1997 Approaches to informed consent. Controlled Clinical Trials 18(6):621–627

Tomamichel M, Sessa C, Herzig S et al 1995 Informed consent for phase I studies: evaluation of quantity and quality of information provided to patients. Annals of Oncology 6: 363–369

Western Consortium for Cancer Nursing Research (1987) Priorities for cancer nursing research. A Canadian replication. Cancer Nursing 10(6):319–326

Wheeler V 1991 Preparing nurses for clinical trials. Seminars in Oncology Nursing 7(4):275–279

World Health Organization Quality of Life Group (1995). The World Health Organization Quality of Life Group assessment: position paper from the World Health Organization. Social Science and Medicine, 41(10):1403–1409

Information and education for patients and families

Emma Ream

7

INTRODUCTION

A cancer diagnosis can elicit shock, disbelief and anger as the patient and family come to terms with news that can bring normal life to a standstill (Hagopian 1993). These natural reactions can serve a protective function. They can allow time for the patient and their family to assimilate the impact of this discovery. However, once the initial shock has abated, patients have to learn a repertoire of new language and skills which will enable them to navigate their way around the hospital, understand diagnostic tests and undergo treatment. Although patients with cancer are frequently admitted to hospital during diagnosis and for the initial stages of their treatment, once their disease is stabilized they generally return home where they manage their symptoms and treatment themselves, or with the support of other family members.

This model of care delivery places the onus on the patient and their family, and reflects the trend in other chronic illnesses for patients to undertake many aspects of their care on a regular or long-term basis (Coates & Boore 1995). Bedell, Cleary & Delbanco (1984) identified four roles that patients have to adopt for this process to be successful, and these appear apposite for patients with cancer. They have to:

1. become aware of activities that impact on healing, and engage in those that enhance their well-being
2. cope with their disease on leaving hospital
3. take an active part in their rehabilitation
4. provide healthcarers with information about their symptoms.

Patients with cancer quickly become aware of the pattern of symptoms caused by their disease and its treatment. For example, after starting chemotherapy, most patients will refer to nadir periods when their blood counts are low and they are susceptible to infections. Or they will mention the risks of nausea and vomiting. What they may be less sure of are the signs and symptoms indicating that they have an infection or are becoming dehydrated, and the steps they should take to deal with them.

If patients with cancer are to become autonomous self-managers of their illness and its treatment, healthcarers have to ensure that they provide them with the knowledge, skills and power to perform this role. The European Working Conference on Cancer Patient Support held in 1991 recognized the importance of education for patients' well-being and placed it in a central position within the declaration of rights that they developed for patients with cancer. This pan-European initiative states patients' right to share in decisions regarding their care and pronounces health professionals' duty to inform patients about their disease in a sensitive manner and to discuss with them their treatment in an honest and informative manner. The declaration emphasizes health professionals' role in help-ing patients, and their family and friends, to understand and come to terms with the cancer diagnosis. Patient education is a crucial aspect of this process, and is in accordance with patients' desire to be involved in decisions about their care (Degner & Russell 1988, National Cancer Alliance 1996).

This chapter will look at the role of information-giving and education in patients' adaptation to living with cancer. It will discuss the benefits for patients of being informed, and consider some theoretical frameworks explaining the relationship between learning and coping. Following this, variables that may act as barriers to patient education, and strategies that nurses can use to optimize educational opportunities, will be discussed. The chapter will conclude with a review of intervention studies that have investigated the effects of education and support on patients with cancer.

INFORMATION AND EDUCATION

The terms information and education are not synonymous with one another. Through providing patients with information, nurses and other healthcare professionals are fulfilling one aspect of their educational role. Health education is a broader process than information-giving, the goals of which are presented below.

Goals of health education (Lipson & Steiger 1996):

- impart information
- help patients to participate effectively in care
- help patients to adjust to the reality of illness and treatment
- help patients to realize the fruits of their efforts.

To achieve these goals, healthcare professionals may need to adopt a broader approach to patient education than that followed traditionally. Although factual information is essential for providing individuals with the necessary knowledge, patients may need practical demonstration to establish the skills required. Furthermore, patients may need encouragement to adopt an unfamiliar relationship with their healthcare team. Rather than being passive recipients of the care prescribed for them, they may need encouragement in becoming partners responsible for aspects of their rehabilitation. Nurses must work to encourage and empower patients to take control for themselves.

BENEFITS OF PATIENT EDUCATION TO PATIENTS WITH CANCER AND THEIR FAMILIES

Over the past 10 years, a number of authors have considered the rationale for, and alluded to, the numerous and varied benefits of education for patients with cancer and their families (Blumberg & Gentry 1991, Fernsler & Cannon 1991, Ganz 1988). Benefits include increased satisfaction, a commonly reported outcome of patient education (Derdiarian 1989), which can be reflected in increased compliance with treatment (Given & Given 1984). Accurate information increases patients' knowledge about the disease and can prepare them for forthcoming investigations and treatment. Patients report less anxiety and distress with medical procedures and treatment when their expectations are realistic and consistent with their actual experiences (Johnson et al 1988). In addition, patients and their families are less distressed by side-effects when they are aware of self-care strategies which they can employ to ameliorate them (Ferrell et al 1995). Self-care, defined as the strategies initiated by patients to enhance their life, health and well-being (Orem 1980), enables patients to participate effectively in their care and exert better control over troublesome side-effects (Dodd 1997). Successful self-care provides patients and their families with a sense of control and mastery (Given & Given 1984). Gaining control over aspects of their care can be particularly pertinent and valuable as patients with cancer frequently report feeling out of control and in the 'lap of the gods' (Ream & Richardson 1997, p. 50).

A further benefit of education for individuals with cancer and their families is their increased mutual understanding of the illness and its prognosis, and the opportunities education provides for families to discuss personal, financial and legal matters. Through mediating and maintaining communication within a family about matters relating to the illness, healthcare professionals can help families to focus as a unit on other matters of concern to them.

Thus, through educating patients and their families about the illness and its treatment, through supporting their efforts to understand it, and welcoming them as partners in their care, healthcare professionals are doing far more than imparting knowledge. They are acting as catalysts, hastening patients' and families' successful adaptation to living with cancer. Through understanding the disease, its effects on their lives and its likely trajectory, patients and their families frequently feel less threatened by it, and more in control of their situation (Fredette & Beattie 1986).

THEORETICAL FRAMEWORKS OF LEARNING AND COPING

Nurses' understanding of the relationship between learning and coping has been furthered by three different theories: self-care theory (Orem 1980), self-regulatory theory (Leventhal, Diefenbach & Guttman 1992, Nerenz & Leventhal 1983) and coping theory (Cohen & Lazarus 1979). These three theoretical frameworks identify the importance of learning in patients' adaptation to illnesses, including cancer. Collectively, they provide a firm theoretical basis on which to base practice and research.

Self-care theory depicts patients as active performers of self-care activities. Self-care activities are those activities undertaken by them which allow them to manage their illness and further their well-being (Orem 1980). Information plays a crucial part in the self-care process, enabling patients to adopt appropriate self-care strategies and retain their independence from healthcare workers. In the initial stages of their illness, for example following surgery, patients may rely completely on the nursing staff, who adopt a fully compensatory role. As time progresses, patients come to understand their illness and measures that can be taken to relieve side-effects and improve quality of life. During this time, nurses undertake a partially compensatory role, performing and explaining procedures, and guiding patients until they master them. When patients return home as autonomous self-managers of their illness, nurses oversee and monitor their progress. Education is a crucial aspect of the self-care process, as without it patients may not be knowledgeable or confident enough to engage in self-care. Self-care theory has guided research into self-care practices of patients with cancer, and the influence of education on the actions that they take (Hagopian 1991, Richardson & Ream 1997).

Cohen & Lazarus (1979) are pioneers of coping theory. Coping has been defined as the constantly changing cognitive and behavioural efforts that individuals employ to manage specific external and/or internal demands which they perceive as taxing or exceeding their personal resources. This theory of coping (there are others, for example Mages & Mendelsohn 1979) proposes that patients adopt coping modes when faced with the stress of illness that either fulfil problem-solving or emotion-regulating functions. Coping efforts can include both behavioural and cognitive elements, according to the challenges of the situation. As a situation changes, or an individual's perception of it alters, the coping mode selected may change. The key aspect is the individual's interpretation of the stressor. Individuals make a judgement about the threat imposed by an event such as contracting cancer (primary appraisal) and form opinions about their ability to control or influence events (secondary appraisal). Their mental representation of their illness will determine the coping strategies that they adopt. Cohen & Lazarus (1979) propose that there are five coping modes that patients adopt to enable them to cope with the emotions engendered by the event or to assert control over the situation. These are:

- information-seeking
- taking direct action
- using intrapsychic defences
- turning to others
- inhibiting action.

Information-seeking is perceived by Cohen & Lazarus as fulfilling a dual function. It can provide the knowledge required for action and, by focusing attention away from the stressful situation at hand, can serve to regulate emotion. Education is fundamental for patients wishing to take direct action, as without it they are unable to understand their illness or take self-care measures to manage it. Stress and coping theory has provided the theoretical basis for nursing research exploring the relationship between preparatory education and the psychological status of patients with cancer, their ability to cope with stress and their satisfaction with their care (Davison, Degner & Morgan 1995, Derdiarian 1989, Poroch 1995).

The final theory that has furthered understanding of the role of education in patients' adaptation to illness is the self-regulatory theory. This theory contends that patients form mental representations of their illness and the meaning that it holds for their life, based on previous experiences, beliefs and expectations (Turk, Rudy & Salovey 1986) acquired throughout their lives, and from new information (Contrada, Leventhal & Anderson 1994). Their perceptions of illness may be inaccurate, perhaps based on ignorance, conjecture and fear. Self-regulatory theory proposes that individuals are more able to adapt to stressful events when their expectations prove realistic when faced with the event. This is more likely when they receive accurate and detailed information. Patients become distressed when their concrete experiences differ from their expectations. Self-regulatory theory has provided a basis for research into preparatory sensory nursing interventions (Johnson et al 1997, Ream, Richardson & Alexander-Dann 1997, Rhodes et al 1994).

Thus, through information and education, patients are more able to develop accurate expectations of their illness and its treatment and to adopt effective self-care strategies to optimize their functioning and well-being. However, there are a number of individual and situational variables that act to make these processes more complex.

INDIVIDUAL VARIABLES

The cancer education literature mentions a number of individual factors that are hypothesized to influence the educational preferences of patients with cancer. For some variables there is more evidence to support these notions than for others. The following section of this chapter discusses the available evidence and, in the absence of firm evidence supporting or refuting the impact of different demographic variables, includes those factors believed to have an influence.

Gender

Anecdotal evidence, and the limited research conducted into the effects of gender on coping and learning, suggests that men react differently to women when faced with a cancer diagnosis. Men express more fear, anger, feelings of depression, despondency and irritability than women (Derdiarian 1987a). The close relationship between adaptation and learning would suggest that these negative cognitions could hinder men's adaptation to their illness, and act as a barrier to their learning. Furthermore, limited research purports that women are more religious than men (Derdiarian 1987a) and find solace in their beliefs, which assists them in coming to terms with the diagnosis. However, although these hypothesized relationships between gender, adaptation and learning have yet to be tested or confirmed systematically, practitioners should be aware that gender may influence the learning needs of patients at different stages of their illness.

Age and developmental stage

Patients' learning needs and ability will change according to their developmental stage. The information and support needed by an adolescent or young adult will be appreciably different from that required by an older adult, or someone nearing retirement. Adolescents are likely to be concerned about their appearance (Enskar et al 1997, Hinds, Quargnentin & Wentz 1992, Ohanian 1990), their status amongst their peers (Faulkener, Peace & O'Keeffe 1995), their fertility and sexuality (Whyte & Smith 1997) and their ability to engage in meaningful relationships with others (Enskar et al 1997). However, their receptiveness to information and support from healthcare professionals may be influenced by their attitudes towards figures of authority. Young adults frequently pass through a stage of rebellion, which may be exacerbated by feelings of anger and vulnerability evoked by the cancer diagnosis. It is not unusual for young adults and children to become difficult to manage and resentful at some stage during their cancer treatment (Eiser & Havermans 1992). This can be reflected in poor compliance with treatment and reliance on alcohol and drugs (Hanna 1993, Tebbi 1993). However, research evidence suggests that, despite the young age and immaturity of children and adolescents, these groups of young people are more able to adapt to the diagnosis, comply with treatment and find communication with their parents easier when they understand the diagnosis and the rationale for their treatment (Eiser & Havermans 1992). In addition, accurate information can ease parental concern and inevitable worries about their child's future. If information is withheld from children they may learn about their condition through 'eavesdropping' and observation, neither of which enables discussion or allows them to discuss their feelings and fears. Withholding information from children can result in them feeling isolated and lonely (Eiser & Havermans 1992). However, educational resources must be developed and selected carefully for this group of young people. Information must be relevant to their needs, interesting to them and written in a style that they find accessible. In addition, as young people may not have the cognitive development required for abstract thought, teaching may be more effective when performed at a concrete and task-oriented level.

The informational needs of more mature adults will vary according to their stage of life. Working individuals may be concerned about maintaining their job, or accounting for their financial needs with early retirement. Others may be preoccupied by the impact of their disease on their children or elderly parents (Rowland 1989). Every patient has unique learning needs, and those caring for them must strive to ascertain what these are. Providing them with information that they already know, or with information that is not relevant to their needs at their stage in life, could result in consternation and irritability, and may prove ineffective

(Galloway et al 1997). Furthermore, patients vary in their intellectual capacity and literacy, and educational materials must be selected to reflect these differences. The topic of literacy, learning and educational materials is covered in more detail later in this chapter.

Some evidence suggests that there is a negative relationship between age and information-seeking, with older people desiring less information and involvement in their care than younger patients with cancer (Cassileth et al 1980, Hopkins 1986).

Personality

There is some evidence to support a hypothesized link between individuals' cognitive styles, or personality traits, and their coping styles when faced with stressful situations (Lev 1992, Suls & Fletcher 1985). People with a high internal locus of control express belief in their ability to control a situation, and are likely to take steps to manage adverse events such as being diagnosed with cancer (Dickson et al 1985). These individuals benefit from understanding their diagnosis and the techniques for managing their symptoms and side-effects. It would seem logical that they would be receptive to information about self-care measures that they could adopt to control their reactions to treatment and improve their well-being.

Conversely, patients with an external locus of control tend to believe that their future rests with fate or powers beyond their personal control or understanding (Dickson et al 1985). These beliefs could impact on their desire for information, and it would seem logical that these individuals would be more passive information-seekers, believing that they personally have little effect over their situation. Certainly, some patients when diagnosed with cancer tend to hand control of their cancer treatment to healthcare personnel (Degner & Russell 1988), whilst others can display limited interest in any information and advice that is provided (Hiromoto & Dungan 1991). However, the limited research that has explored the hypothesized link between personal control and the desire for information has been inconclusive (Brockopp et al 1989).

Limited interest in educational material may also arise when the facts are conveyed in an unsuitable manner for a particular person. Whilst some patients enjoy reading in solitude and consider educational leaflets from cancer organizations essential for their learning, others may find reading difficult and unsuited to their unique needs. Patients who enjoy socializing with others in similar situations may learn more from group work, where there are opportunities for learning through social interaction and the sharing of experiences. The benefits of different educational resources and forums for learning are described in further detail later in this chapter.

Coping style

Individuals respond to stressful situations in unique ways depending on the threat imposed by the event itself, and according to their coping style. Some patients, when diagnosed with cancer, find the discovery too distressing and may use distraction and denial techniques to focus attention away from their situation and allow themselves time to accept its reality. These types of techniques, referred to as avoidant strategies (Suls & Fletcher 1985), contrast sharply with attention strategies where attention is focused directly on, rather than away from, the situation and on methods to counteract it. Information-seeking is one type of attention strategy, where patients actively search for information about their condition and methods to treat it. This type of coping strategy can help patients to construct an accurate understanding of their situation and of effective strategies to manage it, and appears to be favoured by younger patients, by those with high internal locus of control and by those with limited disease (Cassileth et al 1980, Hopkins 1986).

Studies evaluating the efficacy of these approaches have indicated that both can be beneficial. Suls & Fletcher (1985) performed a meta-analysis to synthesize the empirical literature and determine whether one type of coping strategy exceeded the other. Their statistical comparison determined that avoidant strategies prove more beneficial in the short run, allowing individuals to deal with the immediate situation when their resources may be insufficient to cope in a problem-focused manner. However, over the long term, attention strategies enabled more effective adaptation to the stressor. Specifically, Suls & Fletcher identified the first 2-week period as one when avoidance is particularly superior to attention-focusing.

Health and treatment

Patients with cancer frequently find that the multiple effects of the disease process and any associated treatment cause them significant symptom distress (Tishelman, Taube & Sachs 1991). Symptoms including nausea, vomiting, pain, anxiety, fatigue and depression contribute to their feelings of discomfort (Holmes 1991) and can affect patients' attentional processes and their capacity for learning (Cimprich 1992). Classes of drugs including sedatives, steroids and some antibiotics can impair patients' cognitive functioning and prevent retention and recall of information. Cimprich (1992) perceives patients' inability to attend to information as an attentional deficit rather than as a technique for coping. The onset of illness such as cancer requires patients to assimilate large quantities of information about diagnosis, hospital appointments, treatment and side-effects. Frequently this information is imparted over a short period of time, under stressful conditions and at a time when patients are feeling unwell, vulnerable and overwhelmed. At these times they may be unable to concentrate on the information provided by health professionals. They may not retain the information that they are given, as mental effort is required to block out distractions, anxieties and emotions and to maintain the clarity of their thoughts (Cimprich 1992, Wochna 1997). Given the multiple factors that can tax patients' attentional capacity, Cimprich (1992, p. 50) writes that patients with cancer would have 'exceptional demands on direct attentional capacity even under the most favourable circumstances'.

Attentional capacity has particular importance for healthcare professionals who are responsible for informing patients about their diagnosis, available sources of information and support, and future treatment and appointments. The evidence provided suggests that in the immediate period following a diagnosis of cancer, healthcare professionals should be aware that patients may neither want information about their condition nor be able to comprehend and retain it. Careful assessment of patients' educational requirements and preferences at this stage is essential. Care should be taken not to overburden patients with information, and healthcare professionals should concentrate on providing patients with the minimum essential information and provide further more detailed information at a later stage.

Past experience

Individuals' feelings on entering the healthcare system when diagnosed with cancer, and their attitudes towards the healthcare professionals caring for them, will depend in part on their previous experiences. Individuals form their mental representations, or understandings, about life situations from their previous exposure to similar events, either personally or from information they have read or heard (Contrada, Leventhal & Anderson 1994, Turk, Rudy & Salovey 1986). With the taboo and fear associated with cancer (Coughlan 1993), it is not surprising that patients may initially reject efforts by nurses to engage in conversations about the disease. Initial education may need to allay misconceptions about the illness before discussion can progress towards living and coping with the disease.

Education and literacy

The influence of education and literacy on the learning ability of patients with cancer has not been studied to a significant extent. The limited research conducted to date suggests that patients of low socioeconomic status with cancer express more despondency with their situation than those of higher socioeconomic status, and are less assertive than their more affluent counterparts who generally seek more information and medical advice (Derdiarian 1987a). Efforts must be made to ensure that patients have equal access to appropriate information. Patients with lower literacy and socioeconomic status may need more time and assistance in finding the optimal educational material. There are many approaches that health educators can adopt to inform patients and their families about their diagnosis and treatment. Educational media should be selected according to patients' cognitive ability and literacy.

Culture

Healthcare and the role of patient education will vary across Europe, reflecting the ethnic diversity within and across the cultures of the continent. Different cultural beliefs and customs affect populations' perceptions of health and illness, and determine patients' willingness to monitor and manage their disease. In some cultures, health decisions and interventions are made by senior or powerful members of the family network rather than by the individual.

Different cultural groups may require different types of educational programmes or services. Establishing a cross-cultural understanding between healthcare provider and patient is essential. Through conversations with patients and their family members, healthcarers are able to develop their understanding of their patients' cultural beliefs and practices, and develop their educational programmes accordingly. Given the cultural diversity of individuals across Europe, nurses and other healthcare professionals throughout the continent have to adapt the style and content of educational programmes for patients with cancer, such as the European initiative 'Learning to live with cancer' (Grahn 1993) to suit their region of Europe. The language, logic, experience and illustrations in the materials used will need to reflect the language, logic and experience of the population (Doak, Doak & Lorig 1996).

Thus, there are a number of individual factors which in isolation, and more often in conjunction with one another, impact on patients' educational desires and capacity. These are summarized in Fig 7.1.

SITUATION-RELATED VARIABLES

In addition to individual characteristics, situation-related factors operate which can act as a barrier to learning. The environment where education takes place may not always be conducive to learning. Furthermore, those planning and organizing patient teaching may find they have limited resources for the teaching task.

Environment

The environment can be a factor in hospitals that may prevent teaching efforts from being effective. Educators frequently have to teach patients with cancer under testing surroundings. Hospital wards and outpatient departments are generally distracting environments associated with noise and general commotion. Distractions including noise and movement focus attention away from conversation and the topic under consideration. However, unfortunately, these places are where opportunities for nurse–patient teaching arise. If possible, teaching should be scheduled for times or places where distractions are at a minimum.

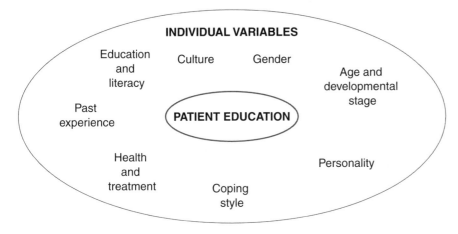

Figure 7.1 Individual variables with an impact on patient education.

Resources

Time is an important commodity for patient teaching. To be effective, patient education must meet patients' needs. It is essential to assess what these are before a teaching strategy is developed. Time is then needed to select the materials before information is conveyed. This process can be lengthy if it is to be successful, and it is easy to underestimate the time that will be involved.

Teaching sessions with patients and their families should be unhurried, and at a speed set by the learners. Throughout the sessions, there should be opportunity to reflect on the new information, to check understanding, answer concerns, and reinforce the message as appropriate. Without time set aside for these reflective purposes, the teaching efforts may fail to meet either the educators' or the learners' expectations.

Educational resources are considered in more detail later in the chapter. However, patient teaching will undoubtedly be influenced by the quality of the materials that are offered to patients. Their appearance, content and detail will affect whether they are read and used by individuals and their families.

Personnel are a key factor in patient education. Nurses with effective communication skills are able to establish a good rapport with patients and families, and identify their information needs (Wochna 1997). Once these are established, a nurse or other healthcare professional with the requisite knowledge of cancer can be involved to answer patients' specific information needs. The communication skills of the person educating the patient are equally important to ensure that the message is conveyed in a sensitive, respectful and honest manner. Research has confirmed that patients favour these characteristics in healthcare professionals discussing their illness, treatment and prognosis (Bliss & Johnson 1993, National Cancer Alliance 1996, Wochna 1997). Patients frequently prefer to be involved in treatment-related decisions (National Cancer Alliance 1996). This is possible when patients feel that their opinions and preferences are valued and valid. Healthcare professionals can create consulting and learning environments that encourage patients to voice their opinions and concerns. These approaches render patients and their families better able to cope with cancer and its treatment, as they foster knowledge about their illness and empower them to manage their illness.

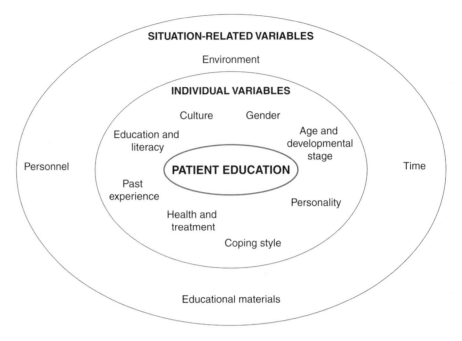

Figure 7.2 Individual and situation-related variables with an impact on patient education.

Thus, situation-related factors can also determine the efficacy of education efforts. A summary of all factors impacting on education is presented in Fig 7.2. Once more, these generally act concurrently, frequently compounding one another, making the educator's role more complex. Educators must take these factors into consideration when planning teaching programmes for patients with cancer and their families, and be aware that these factors determine patients' individual information needs. Some strategies can be employed to ensure that the educational approach taken is suitable for the target audience. These are considered in detail in the next section.

STRATEGIES FOR EFFECTIVE PATIENT EDUCATION

Patient teaching is most successful when it is provided at a time when patients and their families are receptive to teaching, and when the information that is imparted is deemed appropriate, interesting and is presented at the right level. Assessment of learners' needs, preferences and ability to learn are crucial, and teaching programmes should be tailored to suit them. The following section considers assessment of learning preferences, needs and readiness in some depth before discussing strategies to optimize teaching efficacy.

Assessment of learning preferences and needs

Patients with cancer of all ages, gender and socioeconomic status generally express a desire for as much information as possible relating to their disease, prognosis and treatment (Davison, Degner & Morgan 1995, Fallowfield, Ford & Lewis 1995, Hinds, Streater & Mood 1995). However, they frequently report that their information needs are not met and voice dissatisfaction with the information that they receive (Davison, Degner & Morgan 1995, Luker et al 1996). This may be explained in part by the enormous knowledge deficit that most patients face when diagnosed with cancer. Unless they have had previous experience with cancer care services, they find themselves faced with terrifying news in unfamiliar surroundings, where an obscure medical language tends to be spoken. To comprehend fully the implications of a cancer diagnosis for their lives, they may need to acquire an understanding of anatomy, physiology, biochemistry, psychology, and current employment and social security regulations, and so on. It is not surprising that patients refer to feeling overwhelmed at this stage (Cimprich 1992).

Through assessing and prioritizing patients' information needs and incorporating these into a teaching strategy, healthcare professionals can ensure that patients receive the information that they desire during their cancer journey, without being overburdened with facts at any one time – rather more, that information is imparted one step at a time. Models have been developed, including one devised by nurses at the University of Michigan for patients receiving chemotherapy, to assist prioritization of learning needs and development of teaching strategy (Wintermeyer-Pringle et al 1997).

Research suggests that patients' information needs may vary with age (Cassileth et al 1980, Galloway et al 1997, Graydon et al 1997, Hopkins 1986) and education (Cassileth et al 1980). However, these views have been contested by published studies failing to identify such relationships (Fallowfield, Ford & Lewis 1995, Hinds, Streater & Mood 1995), thus confirming the value of individual assessment. Within all groups of patients there will be variability, reflecting the individualistic nature of patients' need for information during the cancer experience, and highlighting the importance of assessing individual need accurately.

The education of patients with cancer and their families is a continual and dynamic process. Their needs and preferences change according to the nature and stage of their illness, their knowledge requirements and their receptiveness to new information. Learning is least likely to be successful if the patient and their family are not ready to learn. Patients and their families progress through a series of psychosocial stages as they adjust to, and cope with, a member of their family contracting cancer. During these different stages their willingness to learn will vary, either as a family unit or individually.

The stage immediately after diagnosis has been considered in detail by Derdiarian (1987a), who used existing theories of coping, needs, appraisal and information-seeking to construct a framework depicting patients' informational needs in these initial stages. In this framework, information is conceived firstly as a mediating factor enabling individuals to appraise the severity of their situation, assess their resources to cope, and identify any knowledge deficit. According to this conception, the need for information is determined by the degree of its lack. Information is deemed relevant and useful when it brings new potential to counteract the perceived threat.

Derdiarian (1987a) reviewed the coping literature for indications of the nature of information required by patients after initial diagnosis. Her systematic search revealed four areas of concern that patients referred to time and again: disease concerns, personal concerns, family concerns and social concerns. Immediately after diagnosis, patients were concerned about the impact of their disease on their immediate and future well-being as an individual, and within their family and social groups. A major concern related to feeling unable to communicate about their diagnosis and maintain relationships with loved ones, peers and colleagues. An additional issue surrounded their ability to continue with work and survive economic implications of ceasing work. These areas, shown in Box 7.1, were identified as those that patients needed information on.

■ **BOX 7.1** **Summary of the information needs of newly diagnosed patients (adapted from the work of Derdiarian 1987a)**

Disease concerns

Impact of disease on survival, specifically:

- diagnosis
- treatment
- tests
- prognosis.

Personal concerns

Impact of disease and treatment on:

- physical well-being and functioning
- psychological and emotional well-being
- job or career
- plans and goals.

Family concerns

Impact of diagnosis on spouse's, children's, parents' and siblings':

- physical well-being
- psychological well-being
- economic well-being
- communication and relationship.

Social concerns

Impact of diagnosis on:

- interaction with peers
- leisure and social interests
- initiation of relationships with other patients and with health professionals.

Influential papers published in the last 5 years support Derdiarian's (1987a) framework of information needs. These papers explore and describe the information needs of specific groups of patients: the needs of men with prostate cancer (Davison, Degner & Morgan 1995); the needs of women at, and following, a diagnosis of breast cancer (Galloway et al 1997, Graydon et al 1997, Luker et al 1995, 1996); and the needs of patients receiving radiotherapy (Hinds, Streater & Mood 1995). Although these groups displayed specific educational requirements relating to their particular diagnosis, they also demonstrated common concerns following diagnosis surrounding the likelihood of cure, the chance of disease progression and the availability of treatment options, suggesting that the information needs of recently diagnosed patients may be universal, relating to their immediate future and well-being. As time progressed, although survival issues remained important, other concerns were raised, including living with cancer and determining the genetic risk of cancer for future generations (Luker et al 1996).

Assessment of patients' individual needs can be aided by questionnaires and needs profiles that have been developed for specific populations. Derdiarian (1987b) developed a generic questionnaire to assess the information needs of patients newly diagnosed with cancer, the Derdiarian Informational Needs Assessment (DINA). This interview instrument has undergone limited psychometric testing with a diverse group of newly diagnosed patients. Although limited, the results of these tests suggest that the DINA could make a valuable contribution in assessing patients with cancer and warrants further testing with further groups of recently diagnosed patients alongside those at different critical stages of living with cancer.

The information needs of women with a recent diagnosis of breast cancer can be identified using self-administered questionnaires including the Toronto Informational Needs Questionnaire – Breast Cancer (Galloway et al 1997) and the Information Preference Questionnaire (Hopkins 1986). Although these questionnaires have not been used widely, initial psychometric testing of the Toronto questionnaire is again favourable (Galloway et al 1997). However, like the DINA (Derdiarian 1987b), these two instruments have been developed and tested solely in American populations, and their cultural relevance for European and other continental populations has yet to be determined. Furthermore, they require time for patients to complete and may be of more benefit as a research instrument than a clinical tool, where need assessment is generally determined through conversation. Evidence from studies employing these instruments can be incorporated into profiles of patient need, describing the information needed by patients at different stages of the disease process to enable them to live with breast cancer and its treatment. An information needs profile of women with breast cancer has been developed in the UK, drawing on available literature; it draws attention to the priority information needs of this patient group (Luker et al 1996). Profiles such as this can be used in clinical settings to guide assessment of the needs of individual women.

Little is known about the information needs of other groups of patients with cancer. Although questionnaires and needs profiles have been developed for women with breast cancer, further research needs to clarify the needs of different patient populations across the disease trajectory. To be effective, information needs to be provided on pertinent areas of concern at the correct time. This cannot be determined without asking patients themselves. Assumptions about patients' educational needs are likely to be inaccurate. The literature is littered with instances where there has been a mismatch between educators' and patients' perceptions of information need (Goldberg et al 1990, Lauer, Murphy & Powers 1982, Pfefferbaum & Levenson 1982).

However, although patients may desire information, they may be unwilling to make treatment-related decisions. This was evident in the study performed by Davison, Degner & Morgan (1995), where the sample of men desired more information than they were given, yet wished to adopt a passive role in their treatment, leaving the management of their prostate cancer to their physicians. In some cases, patients' treatment decisions are guided by their carers and families. Families are an important resource for patients, supporting them through their treatment, helping them gain access to treatment and services, and often bearing the brunt of the physical caring (McDonald, Stetz & Compton 1996). The carer's role is stressful, characterized by isolation, fatigue, economic hardship (when employment is sacrificed) and emotional upset (Jensen & Given 1991). Their educational needs are important and, when fulfilled, they not only enable discussion of treatment options with their relative, but also prepare them for increasing caring responsibilities, which may require complex skills. Complex medication regimens, ambulant chemotherapy and parenteral infusion devices are frequently cared for by family members in the home (Ferrell et al 1995).

However, the educational needs of families are unlikely to be synonymous with, or even reflect, those of the patient (Wochna 1997), and careful assessment of the family unit, in addition to members within it, is crucial. During the last 10 years, research has addressed the educational needs of family caregivers. The data from these studies clarify that family caregivers need information about patients' diagnosis and possible prognosis (Hull 1989, Kristjanson & Ashcraft 1994, Northouse & Peters-Golden 1993, Wochna 1997), the available treatment options and the side-effects associated with them (Kristjanson & Ashcraft 1994, Northouse & Peters-Golden 1993, Wochna 1997) and information on caring for patients at home (Stetz, McDonald & Compton 1996). This information should be tailored, where possible, to meet their needs (Derdiarian 1989, Wochna 1997). These studies have informed the development of educational interventions for family caregivers (Derdiarian 1989, Ferrell et al 1995) and the formulation of recommendations for educating relatives about caring for children receiving chemotherapy (Lilley 1990) and families caring for patients undergoing marrow transplantation (McDonald, Stetz & Compton 1996). These studies draw attention to the quality-of-life benefits for the patient when carers understand the drug treatment, possible side-effects and appropriate interventions.

The different educational needs within families were clearly identified by Ohanian (1990), who conducted research with adolescents and their families. The adolescent patients in this study were concerned with changes in their appearance and feelings of self-worth with the threat of hair loss and infertility, whilst their parents sought information on prognostic indicators. Thus, care must be exercised to ensure that the information needs of the patient, the family as a whole, and of individuals within the family unit are carefully assessed, as their joint and individual needs will change over time. Furthermore, their readiness to learn this information will vary at different stages of the disease and treatment trajectory. The next section considers assessment of learning readiness.

Assessment of learning readiness

Assessment of learning readiness is a fundamental aspect of patient and family education. Before healthcare professionals institute their teaching plan they must be aware of their recipients' willingness to learn about the cancer diagnosis and its implications for their lives. This will be affected by the coping strategies that they are employing to enable them to live with the shattering cancer diagnosis and the uncertainty that it introduces to their lives.

Fredette (1990) explored the existing literature to identify 21 coping strategies that patients employ when faced with serious illness. She proposed that these are exhibited as patients transcend six different adaptive stages during their cancer journey, progressing from initial diagnosis to the terminal period. Fredette suggests that, during this time, patients' receptiveness to information about disease-related matters varies. In the initial periods, characterized by anxiety, dismay and denial, patients will be least receptive to education. As Suls & Fletcher (1985) identified in their meta-analysis, avoidant techniques predominate their coping at this time. As time progresses, and they accept the onset of cancer and its consequences for their lives, patients become open to new ideas and more willing to learn. Suls & Fletcher (1985) identified this period as one when non-avoidant, or attentional strategies, become evident as patients adapt to their illness. These discrete phases provide the basis for Fredette's (1990) educational model for improving education for patients with cancer. Its purpose is to provide a broad framework to guide nursing assessment of patients' learning readiness. This model is especially useful for identifying appropriate teaching strategies across the illness trajectory, corresponding to individuals' and families' readiness to learn. Through adopting such a model, nurses can determine teaching opportunities and target their resources appropriately. A summary of this model is presented in Table 7.1.

The adaptive processes displayed by families of those with cancer are similar to those of patients themselves. Relatives also struggle to make sense of a diagnosis that they may have dreaded, and will vary in their readiness to learn as they strive to understand its implications for the well-being of the patient and the entire family. Although this adaptive process has not been studied to an appreciable extent in children, preliminary evidence suggests that children and adolescents differ in their readiness to learn in a similar manner to adults. Peterson & Toler (1986) showed that children with an inquiring predisposition sought more information before and after surgery than their counterparts. Hence, as with adults, it is important that children's individual desire for information is assessed, and that the materials used to educate them reflect their level of interest and need.

SELECTION OF MEDIA

Patients have greater access to information with the advent of the Internet. Internet support groups, online support groups providing sources of information and psychological support for people with cancer and their families, are increasing (Klemm & Nolan 1998). However, accessibility to information does not necessarily equate with greater understanding, as patients are often confused by the volume and complexity of information they are confronted with (Northouse 1989). Having determined the information priorities at different stages, educators need to select the optimal way of getting their message across. The technological advances in recent years have led to the wide availability of audio and video players and associated educational cassettes, in addition to written educational materials. Although these contribute to patient choice, they may vary in quality and educational content. Care should be exercised in selecting from the range of materials available to find the approach that conveys the message in a meaningful and motivating manner.

Research suggests that before treatment patients prefer information to be conveyed to them on a one-to-one verbal basis by their physician, supported by relevant written material (Hinds, Streater & Mood 1995). The role of the nurse as educator is emphasized after treatment has commenced, when patients require assistance in managing side-effects and adapting to living with cancer (Hinds, Streater & Mood 1995). One-to-one verbal interaction offers patients and their families the opportunity to clarify information, discuss their fears, and obtain the information that they require at that point in time (Hinds, Streater & Mood 1995). It is an expensive approach in terms of physician and nursing time (Meade 1996), and the information is not always retained or understood (Whitman-Obert 1996).

Information booklets and other written materials can reinforce the verbal message and are an accepted means of educating patients about cancer, possible treatment options and potential side-effects. Patients and their families are positive about this educational medium, generally preferring it to audiovisual materials (Hinds, Streater & Mood 1995, Griffiths & Leek 1995). Problems with this approach are encountered in individuals with poor reading skills. Low literacy can prevent patients from understanding and synthesizing written information. Unskilled readers may be able to read words within a passage of text yet fail to grasp the meaning and context of the message (Doak, Doak & Lorig 1996). In these cases, they are unlikely to apply the advice or instructions that are given. This can have enormous implications for patients' management of their cancer treatment at home. Without this understanding, patients and their carers are unlikely to comply with medication regimens, or adopt strategies for the relief of side-effects.

Surveys of materials written for patients with cancer identify their frequent inadequacy. Meade, Diekmann & Thornhill (1992) reviewed the readability of American Cancer Society (ACS) education literature; Cooley et al (1995) considered the readability of ACS and National Cancer Institute materials; Beaver & Luker (1997) surveyed the readability of information booklets for women with breast cancer; and Sarna & Ganley (1995) investigated the availability and quality of patient education materials for patients with lung cancer. All four studies are critical of the readability of the materials. Meade, Diekmann & Thornhill (1992) used the SMOG (Simple Measure of Gobbledygook) reading test to ascertain the general reading level required for the materials and found it to be significantly higher than the average level of reading in the USA. This was subsequently confirmed by Cooley et al (1995). Similarly, the survey within the UK discovered a mismatch between the high reading levels required by the information booklets compared to the reading ability of the population (Beaver & Luker 1997). It was interesting to note that Beaver & Luker reviewed 50 information booklets for women with breast cancer, yet the comparable survey of lung cancer literature (Sarna & Ganley 1995) identified only five educational resources aimed specifically at the needs of this patient group. This illustrates the woeful inequity of information available for different groups, and identifies the difficulty some patients may have in accessing appropriate written information. The five written sources

Table 7.1 Summary of Fredette's model for improving education of the patient with cancer (developed from Fredette 1990)

Adaptation stage	Coping behaviour	Teaching strategy
Exhibiting denial or disbelief	Refusing to acknowledge the diagnosis Diverting attention to other issues Preoccupation with detail	Individual one-to-one teaching Simple concise explanations focused on diagnosis, treatment and impact on life Short frequent teaching sessions
Developing awareness and acceptance of illness	Expressing anger as reality of situation dawns Expressing discouragement Expressing feelings of guilt and depression Deflecting anger at others, appearing impatient, irritable and demanding	Short and frequent one-to-one teaching sessions Identify and enhance useful coping strategies Factual, concise information to dispel guilt and educate about illness and treatment Introduction of written information and simple audiovisual programmes
Moderating thoughts and feelings	Expressing less intense feelings Building and restoring family relationships Accepting dependency on others	Varied as patient and family become more open to new ideas and methods of learning; incorporate leaflets, self-learning programmes, audio and videotapes Group teaching valuable as become more open to sharing Re-teaching to reinforce earlier information
Resolved to illness and accepting changes to self and life	Reassessing image of self and of life with cancer Reordering priorities Acknowledging and accepting changes in themselves and their lives Identifying with others with cancer	Group teaching valuable with acceptance of group identity Information aimed at adaptation to chronic illness Important topic, living as a cancer survivor, i.e. coping with: economic issues, fear of recurrence, treatment of continuing side-effects, stress and interpersonal problems

Decline and deterioration	Expressing denial with progression of disease and institution of palliative care Expressing depression and irritability as physical changes become evident (e.g. anorexia, weight loss and fatigue)	Revert to frequent one-to-one teaching sessions Simple concise explanations focused on interpreting what is happening and choosing treatment Encourage intrafamily communication and support
Terminal phase	Accepting greater dependence on others Yielding responsibility and ceasing self-care For some, expressing denial and rejecting reality of death Vacillating between previous stages of anger, denial, sadness, envy of others, and acceptance	Adopt flexible approach according to adaptive stage and coping behaviour adopted Provide information as issues arise; may include: symptom management, death, grieving, communication problems, and other anxieties and fears Adopt short and frequent one-to-one teaching sessions, coinciding with physiological and psychological comfort Reinforce information and explanations Encourage intrafamily communication and support

identified provided insufficient information, and were again written at levels in excess of those of the American population using them (Sarna & Ganley 1995).

These startling revelations suggest that, although patients find written information of most value, the resources that are available nationally and internationally may be unsuitable for the majority of patients with cancer. Some evidence suggests that in recent years more attention has been paid to simplify written materials on cancer (Meade, Diekmann & Thornhill 1992), but in the absence of adequate resources – nurses have expressed difficulty in obtaining educational resources (Griffiths & Leek 1995) – clinicians may need to create their own. This process is not always successful, as the readability of leaflets designed by nurses more often than not exceeds the reading ability of the intended population (Mumford 1997). Doak, Doak & Lorig (1996) provide useful strategies for improving written cancer education materials. Their guidelines incorporate strategies for optimizing patients' understanding of the message and enhancing their motivation to read and use the material.

Audiocassettes provide a third, and cost-effective, means of conveying cancer education. They are relatively inexpensive to produce and purchase, and can be played many times over. They provide a consistent form of teaching, and patients can learn at their own speed, stopping if they feel saturated, and returning to facts that were unclear. They can be useful supplements to written information, and can be played privately using a Walkman cassette player or in the car. Despite these advantages, audiocassettes have not been used widely and are considered less useful by patients with cancer than conventional written materials (Griffiths & Leek 1995). This attitude may reflect the content and quality of the recorded information rather than the method used to impart the message. Certainly, some groups have derived benefits from taped information. An experiment evaluating informational audiotapes with patients undergoing radiotherapy found them to be an effective approach for teaching self-care strategies in this patient group (Hagopian 1996). Audiocassettes have also been used to record medical consultations, which patients replay in their own time. These serve to remind them of often complex and new information which can prove difficult to recall at a later date. This evidence indicates the value of audiocassettes in certain circumstances. Further research and use in clinical practice will provide more evidence of their efficacy. A word of caution in the meantime: there is evidence to suggest that patients 'switch off' after 15 minutes if they listen to taped information continuously (Babcock & Miller 1993).

Videocassettes are a relatively expensive patient education medium, but the cost can be offset by their potential as an individual or group learning aid. Videotapes can also be effective in saving nursing time (Meade 1996), a benefit that is sometimes overlooked when costs are calculated. Like audiocassettes, videocassettes provide a consistent form of teaching in a medium that is familiar to most patients (Meade 1996). A pertinent and realistic video can capture patients' experiences and enable those viewing it to identify clearly with the characters and scenarios on the screen. This identity can capture interest and help later recall of information. Videotapes can assist in demonstrating self-care strategies to any size of patient group, for example strategies for managing fatigue, dyspnoea and other side-effects. Videotapes can be particularly useful for educating individuals and groups with low literacy skills who find written materials inaccessible (Meade 1996). Patients with cancer have demonstrated enhanced short-term knowledge (Cassileth et al 1982) and reduced anxiety levels (Meade 1996) following educational videos. Videos can also be used in group settings to stimulate discussion and experiential learning. The quality of the video, as with all educational media, will vary and selection should be based on their educational content and presentation style. In the absence of adequate resources, clinicians can produce their own videocassettes.

Meade (1996) covers in detail the process, from planning stages to production and post-production, that is required to produce videotapes for cancer education.

Teaching programmes, including the American programme 'I can cope' (Johnson 1982), 'Living with cancer' (Fredette & Beattie 1986) and, more recently, the European initiative 'Learning to live with cancer' (Grahn 1993), have shown the value of teaching courses aimed at living with cancer. These generic courses, for patients with any cancer diagnosis and their families, allow individuals to attend formal teaching sessions, provide them with written educational materials and provide time for experiential learning through sharing of experience. This multimedia approach has proved beneficial in promoting understanding and mobilizing coping responses. The popularity of multimedia approaches with patients with cancer has been identified by Cooley et al (1995), who found that patients frequently prefer learning approaches that combine more than one method of instruction.

It is likely that patients will view and use a variety of educational materials during their cancer journey. The success of educational programmes will depend to some extent on the materials used to convey the intended message. For some cohorts of patients, notably those with breast cancer, there are extensive resources. For others, including those with lung cancer, the range of materials is limited. Healthcare professionals have to select these resources carefully to ensure that they are understandable, interesting and informative for their intended audience. Materials provided for young people or those from minority ethnic groups must be congruent with their cultural understandings (Boston 1993). If resources are in short supply, educators may have to be innovative with their use, or create their own materials. If possible, clinicians should have access to a range of teaching resources, which can be tailored into teaching programmes to suit individuals' and families' learning styles and needs.

RESEARCH EVALUATING THE EFFICACY OF TEACHING INTERVENTIONS

Numerous studies evaluating the efficacy of patient education for patients with cancer have been published. This research has employed a variety of different designs to investigate the efficacy of educational interventions in differing groups of patients. Educational interventions have been introduced to prepare patients for treatment (Huchcroft et al 1984), to reduce anxiety (Poroch 1995), to improve coping (Fawzy, Fawzy & Wheeler 1996), to enhance self-care (Dodd 1988), to increase knowledge (Dodd 1982) and to improve the management of symptoms and side-effects associated with cancer and its treatment (Hagopian 1991, Rimer et al 1987).

It can be difficult to locate research reports at times, and the findings from studies may be difficult to interpret when they appear inconsistent or contradictory. Fortunately, a number of reviews and meta-analyses, evaluating the efficacy of educational programmes in oncology research, have been published recently. These literature reviews provide a valuable resource for clinicians and researchers alike, providing a résumé of current knowledge and research findings.

Ream & Richardson (1996) performed a traditional review of the literature related to coping with chemotherapy and radiotherapy. They analysed critically the role of information in patients' adaptation. The conclusions of their endeavours confirm the benefits of information in reducing anxiety, enhancing patients' perceptions of control and self-efficacy, and increasing their performance of self-care.

Two meta-analyses of psychosocial (Meyer & Mark 1995) and psychoeducational (Devine & Westlake 1995) interventions in adult patients likewise testify to the

Table 7.2 Summary of the reviews and meta-analyses describing the efficacy of education for patients with cancer

Reference	Type of intervention	Sampling method	Sample size	Findings	Recommendations
Ream & Richardson (1996)	Informational interventions	Sample identified from published multidisciplinary literature	Six studies	Information increased self-care, lowered anxiety and enhanced functioning	Need to: control confounding sociodemographic variables within experiments; quantify the psychological outcomes of information giving; ensure adequate sample size; use consistent interventions and instrumentation
Smith, Holcombe & Stullenbarger (1994)	Symptom management interventions (included patient training and teaching)	Sample identified from published and unpublished nursing research reports, 1981–1990	28 studies	Symptom management relieved symptoms, notably nausea and vomiting, pain, anxiety, alopecia, infection and chemotherapy side-effects	Need: more rigorous experiments to determine the efficacy of symptom management; to use nursing theory as a basis; and to improve research reporting

Devine & Westlake (1995)	Psychoeducational interventions	Sample identified from published and unpublished multidisciplinary literature, 1976–1993	116 studies	Psychoeducational care benefited adults in relation to anxiety, depression, mood, nausea, vomiting, pain and knowledge	Need: more research evaluating the relative efficacy of different psychoeducational care. Clinicians need to examine practice and optimize research-based psychoeducational care
Meyer & Mark (1995)	Psychosocial interventions (included psychoeducational interventions)	Sample identified from published and unpublished multidisciplinary literature, excluded hospice and home care studies	45 studies	Psychosocial interventions benefited emotional adjustment, functional adjustment and symptom/disease-related symptoms	Need: more direct comparison of different treatments; long-term studies of survival time; to investigate ways of increasing the impact of interventions and reducing their cost

statistically significant beneficial effects of education for patients' anxiety, depression, mood, nausea, vomiting, pain and knowledge. These analyses included work from all healthcare disciplines, including medicine, nursing and psychology.

A further meta-analysis synthesized from nursing journals (Smith, Holcombe & Stullenbarger 1994) focused on the effectiveness of nursing interventions for symptom management. This review identified the value of teaching self-care, especially in patients receiving chemotherapy, but identified variations in teaching efficacy with effect sizes ranging from 0.07 (small) to 1.83 (moderate). The authors suggest that this anomaly reflects the different study conditions and interventions incorporated. A summary of the scope and conclusions from these reviews is presented in Table 7.2.

Conclusions evident from these studies indicate that there is a relatively strong research base of intervention studies investigating the effects of education and support on adults with cancer. These investigations recognize the benefits of informing patients about cancer and its treatments, and in training them in strategies including behavioural ones such as relaxation and imagery to enable them to adapt to living with the disease. A combination of education and support can help patients to master the information they need to comply with treatment or recovery programmes. These interventions have benefits for both physical symptoms, including nausea and pain, and the enhancement of emotional well-being, serving to reduce anxiety and depression. The importance of printed materials in this process has been identified (Devine & Westlake 1995), supporting the evidence from previous research (Griffiths & Leek 1995, Hinds, Streater & Mood 1995). The clear message from these studies is not whether education and support are beneficial – they clearly are, with all types of intervention proving effective. The message is rather that nurses need to continue through research to identify the best way to educate and support patients at different stages of their disease, and through clinical practice to explore ways to incorporate teaching interventions into their practice.

CONCLUSION

Health education is undoubtedly desired by patients with cancer and their families, and can assist their adaptation to living with a cancer diagnosis and the treatment that it entails. Education benefits not only the management of physical symptoms but also the learners' psychological and emotional well-being. The importance of education is reflected in recent national and pan-European policy initiatives perceiving education as the patients' right, and something they have every right to expect – for example, the Patients' Charter (Hogg 1986).

Educational programmes for patients with cancer should be developed with care. Consideration should be paid to the timing of information-giving. Patients' physical and psychological status, their symptoms and concentration span should be assessed, along with their motivation and readiness to learn. In addition, the media used to relay the education message should be in tune with their needs, take account of their level of literacy, and reflect their developmental stage and cultural beliefs and practices.

Effective educational initiatives should incorporate a stage of evaluation, where the success of the programme is reflected on. Through looking at outcomes, researchers and clinicians can refine programmes and increase their efficacy. During such evaluation, the relationship between patients, their families and associated healthcare professionals can be assessed to determine the extent to which patients are included as partners in their care, assuming this is what they desire. A further guide to assessing the effectiveness of educational initiatives is provided by Lipson & Steiger (1996) and was discussed at the beginning of this chapter. Patients can be evaluated in terms of their:

1. understanding, knowledge and skills
2. effective participation in care
3. adjustment to the reality of illness and treatment
4. realization of the fruits of their efforts.

The research evaluating the role of education and support in patients' adaptation to cancer confirms their unequivocal value. However, cancer care is a dynamic discipline and healthcarers must ensure that patient education keeps abreast of developments in medical treatment. Patients must be prepared for these changes, and educators must be pro-active – ready and equipped with accurate and relevant information – rather than reactive – developing information in an *ad hoc* and unsystematic manner.

To summarize, there is a relatively substantial theoretical and research base to support the development of teaching initiatives for patients with cancer. This presents three challenges for cancer nurses of the future. The challenge for researchers in the coming months and years lies in building upon the current research base through conducting systematic and rigorous research. It should address current areas of weakness by studying the needs of different patient groups, including children, adolescents, and patients such as those with lung cancer and the majority of other forms of solid or haematological tumours (except those with breast cancer) whose needs have largely been neglected. In addition, research needs to explore further the educational needs of spouses and families. Furthermore, education and support are unequivocally beneficial, and research efforts should now compare different educational approaches within the same study to determine their relative efficacy.

The challenge for clinicians lies in exploring where and how best to incorporate teaching interventions in practice. All too frequently teaching is unplanned and *ad hoc*. The challenge for the entire oncology nursing profession is to increase the impact of educational interventions. Educational interventions have an enormous, and often untapped, potential for patients with cancer that is ready to be harnessed.

REFERENCES

Babcock D, Miller M 1993 Client education theory and practice. Mosby-Year Book, St Louis
Beaver K, Luker K 1997 Readability of patient information for women with breast cancer. Patient Education and Counseling 31:95–102
Bedell A, Cleary P, Delbanco T 1984 The kindly stress of hospitalization. American Journal of Medicine 77:592–596
Bliss J, Johnson B 1993 Cancer patients' perceptions of need. Final report to Cancer Relief Macmillan Fund. King's College London, University of London, London
Blumberg B, Gentry E 1991 Selecting a systematic approach for educating hospitalised cancer patients. Seminars in Oncology Nursing 7(2):112–117
Boston P 1993 Culture and cancer: the relevance of cultural orientation within cancer education programmes. European Journal of Cancer Care 2:72–76
Brockopp D, Hayko D, Davenport W, Winscott C 1989 Personal control and the needs for hope and information among adults diagnosed with cancer. Cancer Nursing 12(2):112–116
Cassileth B, Zupkis R, Sutton-Smith K, March V 1980 Information and participation preferences among cancer patients. Annals of Internal Medicine 92(6):832–836
Cassileth B, Heiberger R, March V, Sutton-Smith K 1982 Effect of audiovisual cancer programmes on patients and families. Journal of Medical Education 57:54–59
Cimprich B 1992 A theoretical perspective on attention and patient education. Advances in Nursing Science 14(3):39–51
Coates V, Boore J 1995 Self-management of chronic illness: implications for nursing. International Journal of Nursing Studies 32(6):628–640

Cohen F, Lazarus R 1979 Coping with the stresses of illness. In: Stone G, Cohen F, Adler N (eds) Health psychology – a handbook. Jossey-Bass, San Francisco, p 217

Contrada R, Leventhal H, Anderson J 1994 Psychological preparation for surgery: marshalling individual and social resources to optimise self-regulation. In: Maes S, Leventhal H, Johnston M (eds) International review of health psychology. John Wiley, New York, vol 3, p 219

Cooley M, Moriarty H, Berger M, Selm-Orr D, Coyle B, Short T 1995 Patient literacy and the readability of written cancer educational materials. Oncology Nursing Forum 22(9):1345–1351

Coughlan M 1993 Knowledge of diagnosis, treatment and its side effects in patients receiving chemotherapy for cancer. European Journal of Cancer Care 2:66–71

Davison B, Degner L, Morgan T 1995 Information and decision-making preferences of men with prostate cancer. Oncology Nursing Forum 22(9):1401–1408

Degner L, Russell C 1988 Preferences for treatment control among adults with cancer. Research in Nursing Health 11(6):367–374

Derdiarian A 1987a Information needs of recently diagnosed cancer patients. A theoretical framework. Part I. Cancer Nursing 10(2):107–115

Derdiarian A 1987b Information needs of recently diagnosed cancer patients. Part II. Method and description. Cancer Nursing 10(3):156–163

Derdiarian A 1989 Effects of information on recently diagnosed patients' and spouses' satisfaction with care. Cancer Nursing 12:285–292

Devine E, Westlake S 1995 The effects of psychoeducational care provided to adults with cancer: meta-analysis of 116 studies. Oncology Nursing Forum 22(9):1369–1381

Dickson A, Dodd M, Carrieri V, Levenson H 1985 Comparison of cancer-specific locus of control and the multidimensional health locus of control scales in chemotherapy patients. Oncology Nursing Forum 12(3):49–54

Doak C, Doak L, Lorig K 1996 Selecting, preparing and using materials. In: Lorig K (ed) Patient education. A practical approach. Sage, Thousand Oaks, California, p 117

Dodd M 1982 Cancer patients' knowledge of chemotherapy: assessment and informational interventions. Oncology Nursing Forum 9(3):39–44

Dodd M 1988 Efficacy of proactive information on self-care in chemotherapy patients. Patient Education and Counseling 11:215–225

Dodd M 1997 Self-care: ready or not! Oncology Nursing Forum 24(6):983–990

Eiser E, Havermans T 1992 Children's understanding of cancer. Psycho-oncology 1:169–181

Enskar K, Carlsson M, Golsater M, Hamrin E 1997 Symptom distress and life situation in adolescents with cancer. Cancer Nursing 20(1):23–33

Fallowfield L, Ford S, Lewis S 1995 No news is good news: information preferences of patients with cancer. Psycho-oncology 4:197–202

Faulkener A, Peace G, O'Keeffe C 1995 When a child has cancer. Chapman Hall, London

Fawzy F, Fawzy N, Wheeler J 1996 A post-hoc comparison of the efficiency of a psychoeducational intervention for melanoma patients delivered in a group versus individual formats: an analysis of data from two studies. Psycho-oncology 5(2):81–89

Fernsler J, Cannon C 1991 The whys of patient education. Seminars in Oncology Nursing 7(2):79–86

Ferrell M, Grant M, Chan J, Ahn C, Ferrell B 1995 The impact of cancer pain education on family caregivers of elderly patients. Oncology Nursing Forum 22(8):1211–1218

Fredette S 1990 A model for improving cancer patient education. Cancer Nursing 13(4):207–215

Fredette S, Beattie H 1986 Living with cancer. A patient education program. Cancer Nursing 9(6):308–316

Galloway S, Graydon J, Harrison D et al 1997 Informational needs of women with a recent diagnosis of breast cancer: development and initial testing of a tool. Journal of Advanced Nursing 25(1):1175–1183

Ganz P 1988 Patient education as a moderator of psychological distress. Journal of Psychosocial Oncology 6(1/2):181–197

Given B, Given C 1984 Creating a climate for compliance. Cancer Nursing 7(2):139–147

Goldberg R, Guadagnoli E, Silliman R, Glicksman A 1990 Cancer patients' concerns: congruence between patients and primary care physicians. Journal of Cancer Education 5:193–199

Grahn G 1993 'Learning to cope' – an intervention in cancer care. Supportive Care in Cancer 1:266–271

Graydon J, Galloway S, Palmer-Wickham S et al 1997 Information needs of women during early treatment for breast cancer. Journal of Advanced Nursing 26(1):59–64

Griffiths M, Leek C 1995 Patient education needs: opinions of oncology nurses and their patients. Oncology Nursing Forum 23(9):139–144

Hagopian G 1991 The effects of a weekly radiation therapy newsletter on patients. Oncology Nursing Forum 18(7):1199–1203

Hagopian G 1993 Cognitive strategies used in adapting to a cancer diagnosis. Oncology Nursing Forum 20(5):759–763

Hagopian G 1996 The effects of informational audiotapes on knowledge and self-care behaviours of patients undergoing radiation therapy. Oncology Nursing Forum 23(4):697

Hanna K 1993 Health behaviours of adolescents who have been diagnosed with cancer. Issues in Comprehensive Pediatric Nursing 16(4):219–228

Hinds P, Quargnentin A, Wentz T 1992 Measuring symptom distress in adolescents with cancer. Journal of Pediatric Oncology Nursing 9:84–86

Hinds C, Streater A, Mood D 1995 Functions and preferred methods of receiving information related to radiotherapy. Cancer Nursing 18(5):374–384

Hiromoto B, Dungan J 1991 Contract learning for self-care activities. Cancer Nursing 14(3):148–154

Hogg C 1986 Patients' charter guidelines for good practice. Association of Community Health Councils for England and Wales, London

Holmes S 1991 Preliminary investigations of symptom distress in two cancer patient populations: evaluation of a measurement instrument. Journal of Advanced Nursing 16(4):439–446

Hopkins M 1986 Information-seeking and adaptational outcomes in women receiving chemotherapy for breast cancer. Cancer Nursing 9(5):256–262

Hull M 1989 Family needs and supportive nursing behaviours during terminal cancer. A review. Oncology Nursing Forum 16:787–792

Huchcroft S, Snodgrass T, Troyan S, Wares C 1984 Testing the effectiveness of an information booklet. Journal of Psychosocial Oncology 2(2):73–83

Jensen S, Given B 1991 Fatigue affecting family caregivers of cancer patients. Cancer Nursing 14(4):181–187

Johnson J 1982 The effects of a patient education course on persons with a chronic illness. Cancer Nursing 5(2):117–123

Johnson J, Nail L, Lauver D, King K, Keys H 1988 Reducing the negative impact of radiation therapy on functional status. Cancer 61:46–51

Johnson J, Fieler V, Wlasowicz G, Mitchell M, Jones L 1997 The effects of nursing care guided by self-regulation theory on coping with radiation therapy. Oncology Nursing Forum 24(6):1041–1050

Klemm P, Nolan M 1998 Internet cancer support groups: legal and ethical issues for nurse researchers. Oncology Nursing Forum 25(4):673–676

Kristjanson L, Ashcraft T 1994 The family's cancer journey. A literature review. Cancer Nursing 17:1–17

Lauer P, Murphy S, Powers M 1982 Learning needs of cancer patients: a comparison of nurse and patient perceptions. Nursing Research 31(1):11–16

Lev E 1992 Patients' strategies for adapting to cancer treatment. Western Journal of Nursing Research 14(5):595–617

Leventhal H, Diefenbach M, Guttman M 1992 Illness cognition: using commonsense to understand treatment adherence and affect cognition reactions. Cognitive Therapy and Research 16:143–163

Lilley L 1990 Side effects associated with pediatric chemotherapy: management and patient education issues. Paediatric Nursing 16(3):252–255

Lipson J, Steiger N 1996 Self-care nursing in a multicultural context. Sage, Thousand Oaks, California

Luker K, Beaver K, Leinster S, Owens R, Degner L, Sloan J 1995 The information needs of women newly diagnosed with breast cancer. Journal of Advanced Nursing 22(1):134–141

Luker K, Beaver K, Leinster S, Owens R 1996 Information needs and sources of information for women with breast cancer: a follow up study. Journal of Advanced Nursing 23:487–495

Mages S, Mendelsohn R 1979 Effects of cancer on patients' lives: a personological approach. In: Stone G, Cohen F, Alder N et al (eds) Health psychology – a handbook. Jossey-Bass, San Francisco, p 255

McDonald J, Stetz K, Compton K 1996 Educational interventions for family caregivers during marrow transplantation. Oncology Nursing Forum 23(9):1432–1439

Meade C 1996 Producing videotapes for cancer education: methods and examples. Oncology Nursing Forum 23(5):837–846

Meade C, Diekmann J, Thornhill D 1992 Readability of American Cancer Society patient education literature. Oncology Nursing Forum 19(1):51–55

Meyer T, Mark M 1995 Effects of psychosocial interventions with adult cancer patients: a meta-analysis of randomized experiments. Health Psychology 14(2):101–108

Mumford M 1997 A descriptive study of the readability of patient information leaflets designed by nurses. Journal of Advanced Nursing 26:985–991

National Cancer Alliance 1996 Patient centred cancer services: what patients say. NCA, Oxford

Nerenz D, Leventhal H 1983 Self-regulation theory in chronic illness. In: Burish T, Bradley L, (eds) Coping with chronic disease – research and applications. Academic Press, New York, p 217

Northouse L 1989 The impact of breast cancer on patients and husbands. Cancer Nursing 12(5):276–284

Northouse L, Peters-Golden H 1993 Cancer and the family: strategies to assist spouses. Seminars in Oncology Nursing 9:74–82

Ohanian N 1990 Cancer patients and their families. Journal of Paediatric Oncology Nursing 7(2):63–64

Orem D 1980 Nursing: concepts and practice, 2nd edn. McGraw-Hill, New York

Peterson L, Toler S 1986 An information seeking disposition in child surgery patients. Health Psychology 5:343–358

Pfefferbaum B, Levenson P 1982 Adolescent cancer patient and physician responses to a questionnaire on patient concerns. American Journal of Psychiatry 139:348–351

Poroch D 1995 The effect of preparatory patient education on the anxiety and satisfaction of cancer patients receiving radiotherapy. Cancer Nursing 18(3):206–214

Ream E, Richardson A 1996 The role of information in patients' adaption to chemotherapy and radiotherapy: a review of the literature. European Journal of Cancer Care 5:132–138

Ream E, Richardson A 1997 Fatigue in patients with cancer and chronic obstructive airways disease. International Journal of Nursing Studies 34(1):44–53

Ream E, Richardson A, Alexander-Dann C 1997 Patients' sensory experiences before, during and immediately following the administration of intravenous chemotherapy. Journal of Cancer Nursing 1(1):25–31

Rhodes V, McDaniel R, Hanson B, Johnson M 1994 Sensory perception of patients on selected antineoplastic chemotherapy protocols. Cancer Nursing 17(1):45–51

Richardson A, Ream E 1997 Self-care behaviours initiated by chemotherapy patients in response to fatigue. International Journal of Nursing Studies 34(1):35–43

Rimer B, Levy M, Keintz M, Fox L, Engstrom P, MacElwee N 1987 Enhancing cancer pain control regimes through patient education. Patient Education and Counseling 10:267–277

Rowland J 1989 Developmental stage and adaptation: adult model. In: Holland J, Rowland J (eds) Handbook of psycho-oncology. Psychological care of the patient with cancer. Oxford University Press, New York, p 25

Sarna L, Ganley B 1995 A survey of lung cancer patient-education materials. Oncology Nursing Forum 22(10):1545–1550

Smith M, Holcombe J, Stullenbarger E 1994 A meta-analysis of intervention effectiveness for symptom management in oncology nursing research. Oncology Nursing Forum 21(7):1201–1210

Stetz K, McDonald J, Compton K 1996 Needs and experiences of family caregivers during marrow transplantation. Oncology Nursing Forum 23(9):1422–1427

Suls J, Fletcher B 1985 The relative efficacy of avoidant and nonavoidant coping strategies. Health Psychology 4(3):249–288

Tebbi C 1993 Treatment compliance in childhood and adolescence. Cancer 71(10 suppl):3441–3449

Tishelman C, Taube A, Sachs L 1991 Self-reported symptom distress in cancer patients: reflections of disease, illness or sickness. Social Science and Medicine 33(11):1229–1240

Turk D, Rudy T, Salovey P 1986 Implicit models of illness. Journal of Behavioural Medicine 9(5):453–474

Whitman-Obert H 1996 Patient information handouts: taking care of yourself – a self-help guide for patients with cancer. Oncology Nursing Forum 23(9):1443–1446

Whyte F, Smith L 1997 A literature review of adolescence and cancer. European Journal of Cancer Care 6(2):137–146

Wintermeyer-Pringle S, Estes J, Cimprich B, Marciniak K 1997 Model allows nurses to prioritize patient teaching for chemotherapy. Oncology Nursing Forum 24(3):456–457

Wochna V 1997 Anxiety, needs, and coping in family members of the bone marrow transplant patient. Cancer Nursing 20(4):244–250

Some ethical issues in cancer nursing

P. Anne Scott Yvonne Willems-Cavalli

CHAPTER 8

INTRODUCTION

In this chapter some ethical issues will be raised that are of interest and relevance to cancer nursing. As a starting point, some snapshots of practitioner–patient or practitioner–relative interaction will be examined. Some possible assumptions upon which these particular interactions are based will also be identified. In doing so, attention will be drawn to a number of relevant ethical issues. To discuss the ethical implications of these interactions, an outline will be given of theoretical approaches that may be used to analyse the ethical impact of particular courses of action. The principles of respect for persons, beneficence, non-maleficence and justice are portrayed as useful components of a moral safety net. However, the additional elements of moral interaction, such as moral strategy and role enactment, are also argued to be of particular significance in the ethics of healthcare practice, and in the nursing of patients with cancer in particular. The example of phase 1 clinical trials is used as the context in which a number of these issues combine to produce an ethically difficult situation from the perspective of both patient and practitioner.

INCIDENTS FROM PRACTICE

Situation 1

Nurse to patient's daughter: 'How much does your father know? What has Mr X told him?'

Situation 2

Junior doctor to patient's brother and sister-in-law: 'Depending on how she gets on, we might allow Margaret out for a few hours – or even a weekend.'

Situation 3

Nurse and colleague to close friend of patient: 'Helen seems to be coping, Janice, but she is not talking about what's happened to her – her mastectomy – at all.

The above snippets of conversation, which come directly from incidents in the clinical experience of one of the authors (P.A.S.), indicate that certain assumptions are being made by the healthcare practitioners involved. In the first situation, the staff nurse appears to assume the following: (1) the doctor or surgeon has spoken openly to the daughter; (2) either together with the daughter, or on his or her own initiative, the surgeon has decided to tell the patient some or all of the details of the problem and prognosis; (3) the daughter is fully aware of the conversation that has taken place between the surgeon and the patient; (4) the most appropriate means of the nurse gaining insight into what the patient knows is to ask the daughter, rather than the surgeon or patient; and (5) the staff nurse assumes that the daughter will give a full and accurate account to her, thus potentially setting up a relationship of collusion with a relative, which may or may not work to the patient's benefit.

Clearly, a number of ethical concerns materialize from such a situation. For example, why does the nurse wish to find out what the surgeon has told the patient, or how much the patient knows? Is this simply an invasion of the patient's privacy or is it to help the nurse gain some understanding of the patient? If we assume that the nurse seeks this information to help her understand the patient and how he might perceive his situation, is a relative (in this case the patient's daughter) the best source of the information? A relative might indeed be such a source if, for example, the patient was unconscious or could not communicate, or could communicate only with difficulty. A relative may also fulfil such a function if the patient evidently relies on this family member, trusts the particular individual, and has indicated to staff that he does not wish to be burdened with decisions regarding care and treatment – that the specified relative will take care of things.

In situation 2, the assumption appears to be that once the patient has entered a healthcare institution his or her rights to self-determination and decision-making are relinquished. Apparently these rights pass automatically to the healthcare team whose care the patient is under. Also, there is, implicitly, the assumption that relatives have no influence on, or interest in, decisions regarding the place where their loved one receives care. Observations regarding how the patient (Margaret) is getting on also seem to have a purely medical basis. As in the first situation, a number of important ethical issues are raised in this situation. These issues are to do with patient autonomy, empowerment and appropriate systems of support. Advocacy and who decides what is best for a patient are also an issue.

Situation 3 continues the theme of support systems, and introduces assumptions regarding normal patterns of response in situations of crisis. The nurse does seem to suggest that because the patient is not talking to her, or perhaps to the ward staff, regarding her mastectomy or her cancer, then, clearly, she is not coping, despite appearances. There is perhaps an element of professional megalomania here. The assumption appears to have been made that if the patient is not sharing her psychological distress with staff, then she is denying her ordeal. Such denial is pathological. It seems that confiding in friends or family to the exclusion of healthcare staff, who after all are often complete strangers, is not a possible and reasonable response. Again, issues of patient privacy, autonomy and acceptable behaviour are raised here.

The above discussion indicates that each human situation needs to be considered within its own particular context. There is unlikely to be a simple formula that, once applied, will provide a neat clear answer. This is as true of ethical issues as it is of many other human issues. However, this does not mean that there is no guidance available to help practitioners deal with ethically troubling human situations. What we have attempted to do in the above exposition is to indicate that in healthcare practice, as in most other human activities, the practitioner works from a number of assumptions. To begin to consider one's actions, decisions and practice from an ethical perspective, it is necessary to identify and consider these assumptions. Once the assumptions have been made explicit, they can be examined against certain criteria, in order to determine their ethical appropriateness.

The question regarding who determines such criteria is both interesting and, at the same time, problematic. Much has been written in the field of healthcare ethics over the past 30 years, on both sides of the Atlantic. Much of this literature has roots in two, or increasingly three, philosophical theories: Kantian duty-based theory, utilitarianism and, increasingly, virtue theory. An exposition of these various ethical positions is not within the scope of this chapter. However, a brief description of each may be useful in order to provide a context and framework within which to consider the issues raised in this chapter.

POSSIBLE THEORETICAL APPROACHES

Kantian ethical theory provides a rich and complex framework within which to consider matters of moral interest. For Kant, the only morally pure motivation is duty (Kant 1991). The good person is the person who works from the demands of duty, rather than from self-interest or any similar motive. Kant also claims that the demands of duty are categorical. They must be obeyed. For example, one *must* tell the truth, rather than one should tell the truth if one wants affection and so on.

Two tenets of Kantian theory are of particular interest in healthcare practice. These are the principle of respect for persons and the principle of universalizability. The principle of respect for persons is central to Kantian ethical theory. By this, Kant claims that duty demands that persons are treated as ends in themselves and never merely as means to an end. The principle of universalizability suggests one must act in such a way that one would wish it to became a universal law. Thus, if I do X in situation A, then all others in situation A should also do X. This is an attempt to prevent the moral agent from making an exception of him or herself. In other words, it is an attempt to ensure fairness in moral activity.

The utilitarian position can be seen as an attempt to support the universalizability principle and also help to cope with some of the limitations of Kantian theory. For example, a charge that can be levelled at Kantian theory is that Kant does not tell us what to do when there is a conflict of principle, for example when telling the truth to a patient (or member of staff) conflicts with one's duty to one's family? In its classical form (Mill 1993), utilitarianism hinges on a single principle which demands that in any situation one should do that which will increase benefits over burdens (or increase happiness over pain). Thus, in the above example, where telling truth to a patient conflicts with duty to one's family, the utilitarian will calculate which action will result in greatest net benefit – telling the truth to the patient or fulfilling one's duty to one's family – and will then act accordingly.

Aristotelian virtue theory recognizes the value of rules and principles as guides to action or rules of thumb (Aristotle 1980). However, of greater significance is the development of enduring traits of character, which will ensure that the agent recognizes the good in a specific situation and acts according to this knowledge. Aristotle describes a protracted, staged approach to the development of the virtues, the success of which is grounded in a good upbringing with the appropriate experiences and education.

Following concerns with upbringing and early socialization, Aristotle focuses on the notion of habituation as being an important stage in becoming virtuous. If a person develops the habit of doing certain things, eventually doing the thing becomes second nature. Aristotle suggests that the correct habits of virtuous acts are developed by observing people of virtue and by developing the habits of doing as they do. Traditionally, the training of nurses and doctors contains large elements of apprentice-type training (Ford & Walsh 1994). Therefore, the importance of this notion of habituation will not be lost to either profession. Many of the skills required in nursing and medicine are developed by on-the-job observation and repetitive practice of what seniors have been observed doing.

In terms of becoming morally good or virtuous, Aristotle stresses that it is by learning the habits of the virtuous that one is on the road to achieving moral virtue oneself. In terms of morally sensitive, humane and compassionate practice, one of the most serious failures in nursing and medicine is the general failure within the professions, and among their educators, to identify *role models* in clinical practice who would provide students with the ideals of practice, which Aristotle's virtuous person provides for the student of a virtuous life. An Aristotelian approach to healthcare ethics could help to focus the minds of the nursing profession (or indeed the medical profession) and the profession's educators on the need to identify ethically sensitive role models (i.e. role models who are sensitive to the ethical dimension of nursing practice) for students in the profession, so that desirable habits of practice are encouraged early in the training of practitioners. If this occurs, the character traits that are being suggested in the literature as desirable in the healthcare practitioner, for example compassion, may begin to emerge on something more than an *ad hoc* basis.

A further aspect of Aristotelian theory which seems of importance to healthcare practitioners regards the roles that Aristotle argues are played by emotion and perception in moral insight and action. Traditionally, the nursing ethics literature and education programmes seem heavily influenced by Kantian duty-based theory (e.g. Edwards 1996, Rumbold 1986, Scott 1998). Kant pays scant attention to the role of emotions, seeing them as non-rational and therefore to be kept under the control of reason in moral action and judgement. However, many would argue that moral perception itself is based in an emotional response. If this is allowed, and if Aristotle is correct in supposing that the emotions can be educated, it follows that Aristotle's insight into the need to educate the emotions is a vitally important facet of moral education.

It is from such theoretical roots that criteria which help to determine ethically appropriate behaviour have been worked out within the Western healthcare context. The appropriateness of the approach to healthcare ethics offered by the above principle-based theories (i.e. Kantianism and utilitarianism, sometimes referred to as principlism) has been severely criticized over the past 10 years. In an analysis of the arguments put forward by a number of critics of a principle-based approach, DuBois, Hamel & O'Connell (1994, p. 16) state:

'The similarities and differences among the various approaches to bioethics lead us to an unavoidable conclusion: the moral dimensions of human experience cannot be captured by a single approach. The approaches to bioethics that we explore here are different paths to a common ground. Each method aims at unpacking the dense layers of human experience in an effort to achieve shared insight and to promote informed action. Each in its own way suggests that, although principlism is valuable, it also has serious limitations. This is not surprising since the breadth and depth of human experience will always exceed the reach of any single philosophical or theological system. The similarities and differences between and among phenomenological, hermeneutic, narrative, virtue-based, and casuistic approaches to bioethics underscore the need for a variegated approach to ethical dilemmas.'

None the less a viable alternative, with roots in virtue theory or elsewhere, has yet to be articulated in detail. The position taken by the present authors is that virtue theory has much potential to provide useful guidance to healthcare practitioners (for arguments in support of our position, see Scott 1993, 1995a). However, in Aristotelian fashion, this is not to recommend the withdrawal of attention from the rules and principles derived, for example, from Kantian ethics and/or utilitarianism, if for no other reason than that they may provide a useful moral safety net. Some of the principles constitutive of the moral safety net will be discussed below. Given the time it may take to identify appropriate virtues for the healthcare practitioner, and the thought needed to design appropriate education, a moral safety net may be all that can be hoped for at the present time.

ETHICAL PRINCIPLES

The set of principles most frequently cited in the healthcare ethics literature involve the following: respect for persons, beneficence, non-maleficence and justice (classically described by Beauchamps & Childress 1989). These principles continue to form the basis of ethics teaching and basic ethics texts for many doctors and nurses (e.g. Downie & Calman 1996, Edwards 1996). Although the principle-based approach to issues in healthcare ethics has undoubted limitations, it does not seem an inappropriate place to begin our discussion of the ethical dimension of cancer nursing practice.

Let us return to situation 1 outlined at the beginning of this chapter (p. 161). Why might one be concerned regarding the nurse's action? Perhaps the nurse is motivated by the principles of beneficence and non-maleficence. The nurse may, for example, be trying to understand how the patient sees his situation, and she may wish to avoid distressing the patient by asking painful questions. In this situation, might the nurse's action be considered not only appropriate, but in fact a morally good act? As indicated above, in certain circumstances this might indeed be the case. However, in order to make this judgement one would need to know more of the situation. In particular, one would wish to be sure that the patient's wishes, desires and rights were not being ignored. One would also want to be assured that the nurse was trying to determine what was in the patient's interests rather than what would save the nurse from a sticky encounter with either the patient, or indeed the surgeon.

There is an abundance of empirical research which indicates that healthcare practitioners avoid communication with patients, regarding the patient's condition or prognosis, because they are uncomfortable with such communication (e.g. Lundt & Neale 1987, Seale 1989, Meredith et al 1996). Such communication is normally deemed to be an element of psychosocial care. If we have sound reason to believe that an important part of our care for patients with cancer is psychosocial care, then it would appear that, as registered practitioners who are paid to care for patients with cancer, we have both a professional and a moral duty to be ready to provide this psychosocial support, should our patients need and want it.

This latter point regarding needing and wanting care is important. We may think that a patient needs psychological support, for example. The patient may think otherwise. If this patient is competent then, despite one's own feelings about the matter, this patient has the right to accept therapeutic contact, in Morse's sense of the word, and to refuse anything further (Morse 1991). A practitioner does not have the right to assume that every patient wants or indeed needs psychosocial, spiritual, or any other kind of support or care, apart from that directly or indirectly sought, merely because the patient has a diagnosis of cancer. To assume otherwise offends against the basic Kantian principle of respect for persons. Basic norms of social behaviour have identifiable patterns of interaction when people first meet one another, and as the acquaintance develops. These are often culturally specific. The healthcare environment – the context of healthcare – has its own norms. However, with the growth of consumerism and increasing individualism in Western capitalist society, the healthcare professions are becoming increasingly aware that the traditional norms of healthcare practice, underpinned as they are by paternalism, are no longer wholly acceptable (Bandeman & Bandeman 1995). The perception is that traditional norms need to be rebalanced in the direction of normal social interaction by recognizing not only the knowledge and authority of the practitioner, but also the right to respect of all and the right to autonomy of many of our patients. Thus, what a practitioner may deem good or harmful for me, I may deem the opposite or less of an evil than it would appear. This is because it is my life that is being considered, and I am likely to have greater insight into what is good or harmful for me than an outsider will have, no matter how knowledgeable or well intentioned. Therefore, in order to care effectively for patients, the practitioner must pay them the basic respect of talking to them to try to gain some relevant insight into their perceptions and context. Without this, care may at best be less effective than it otherwise might be, while at worst it may be harmful through negligence.

The snippets of conversation from situations 2 and 3 quoted on page 161 are also of concern in terms of basic respect for the person who is the patient. The extract of conversation used in situation 2 comes from a case scenario (Scott 1999). In this scenario, as indicated above, the junior doctor assumes that visits to family, whether for a few hours or overnight, or even discharge, is of no consequence to Margaret or her family. This is based on a completely paternalistic position, which does not recognize that the patient will have wishes and desires and has a right to have these considered. This right can be argued for from a Kantian perspective of respect for persons, or indeed from a rule utilitarian perspective (Beauchamps & Childress 1989, Smart 1973).

The statement expressed in situation 3 also offends against the patient's autonomy. Here the nurse assumes that unless Helen spills out all her anguish, fear and pain to this nurse, or at least to a member of the nursing staff, then, despite appearances, Helen is not really coping with her illness. The idea that Helen may have close family or friends who in fact are more appropriate confidants and sources of support for her does not seem to have occurred to this nurse. One of the problems with this approach is that it may lead to Helen receiving inappropriate care. She may be the recipient of distressing probing, embarrassing conversations, unnecessary medication and/or referrals and consultations.

What appears to be at issue in this case is the difference between the following two assumptions: (1) that all patients will react in manner A and require intervention X, and (2) that some patients are likely to react in manner A, and are likely to need intervention X.

The means to finding out whether this particular patient is reacting in manner A and requires intervention X is by offering constructive care (Scott 1995b). By constructive care we mean care that is patient focused rather than practitioner focused. This approach to care includes speaking with the patient, and attending fully to the patient, in an attempt to learn the extent of care and support that this particular patient needs, and which is within the nurse's remit to provide.

CONSTRUCTIVE CARE

It is within the context of constructive care, we suggest, that one faces the limits of a principle approach to healthcare ethics. The basic principles of respect, doing good, doing no harm, and justice are likely to be necessary to sound cancer nursing practice. We would also argue, however, that they are not sufficient. In cancer care, as in many other acute and chronic care contexts, nurses have contact with patients who are vulnerable, distressed and frightened of what the future holds for them. How one is with the patient is often as important to the patient as what one does (Carr-Hill & Dixon 1992). It is important, for example, what information the patient receives (Bok 1984). It is also important, however, how that information is given (Randall & Downie 1996). Within the context of a principle-based approach, it is difficult to talk about this dimension of care. Downie (1964), writing on social ethics, articulated the notions of role enactment (how one is in one's role) and moral strategy (the strategies one uses in moral activities). It has been argued elsewhere that these notions are fundamentally important when considering the ethics of healthcare practice (Scott 1995c, 1997). This is based on a particular view of the meaning of healthcare ethics – its field of concern. Following Aristotle, we see ethics as being of practical relevance. We suggest that one of the primary reasons for raising ethical awareness among practitioners, or for teaching healthcare ethics, is to help the practitioner to be a better practitioner, in the sense of being more humane, compassionate, and so on. Perhaps the following two quotes may give some insight into what we see as the multifaceted nature of healthcare ethics:

> *'Ethics is concerned not only with what a certain individual considers right but with what is right. Ethics not merely describes moral ideals held by human beings, but asks which ideal is better than others, more worth pursuing and why ... Perhaps doing right is more important than discovering what right is. But at least the second is a necessary means to the first. Unless you first know what is right, how will you know what to do or what to persuade others to do? ... Acting in moral matters without knowledge is surely as dangerous as trying to build a bridge without knowing the principles of engineering ...' Hospers (1961).*

Again focusing on the ethical importance of the ordinary and everyday inter-action, Martha Levine comments:

> *'Ethical behaviour is not the display of moral rectitude in times of crises. It is the day to day expression of one's commitment to other persons and the ways in which human beings relate to one another in their daily interactions. The very nature of nursing makes it impossible ... to stand aside from the experience of interacting with other human beings. Nursing has a moral responsibility to be as good as education and self awareness can make it be ... only intense personalised involvement can create the moral environment in which care is ... a true response to human need' Levine (1977, p. 845).*

Hospers (1961) focuses the mind on the need to be clear about the meaning of the concepts that we use. This is as important in moral matters as it is in any other important human activity, and has crucial importance for the manner in which we, in our literature and our practice, analyse and conceptualize value-laden notions such as care. Much scholarly work is needed in nursing to develop the conceptual basis of our practice. However, we suggest that it is within the context of Levine's definition that the need to consider notions of role enactment and moral strategy is seen most clearly. If we do not attempt to come to grips with these two notions, particularly within the context of cancer nursing, we will remain at the moral safety net end of nursing and healthcare, and we will fail to care constructively for many of our patients. Because of their potential vulnerabilities, patients with cancer seem at high risk in this regard.

CANCER NURSING AND ETHICAL CONCERNS

In the sections above, consideration has been given to some of the broad, general ideas regarding the place of ethical thinking, language and understanding within the context of cancer nursing. Some of the ethical concerns with which nurses are often confronted in their daily activity will now be addressed. There is, of course, an almost unlimited list of issues that could be discussed here. To do this in some detail is clearly impossible within the limits of this chapter. We choose, therefore, briefly to address only three types of issue and then to discuss in depth the question of how patients with cancer should be informed. In fact, information is a key aspect related to all ethical issues, both regarding its content as well as the very existence of an 'open information channel' between patients and health professionals.

Approaching the patient confronted with cancer

The first item relates to how nurses should react to the attitude of patients con-fronted with cancer. It is well known that there is a huge array of potential emotional reactions, stretching from simple denial of the disease to the most devastating despair. It is also evident that the attitude of most patients will evolve during the course of the disease, generally depending (but not always) on the outcome of the treatment. Taking all this into account, it is quite clear that there is no place for one schematic approach that nurses may follow to assist them in dealing with the emotional attitudes of patients with cancer. On the contrary, nurses and the whole multiprofessional team should learn to analyse the psychosocial background of every patient, while furthermore being able to understand which of the emotional reactions of patients are determined by the specific moment in the course of their disease (diagnosis, hope for cure, deception for negative results or relapse, etc.) (Morse & Doberneck 1995).

While these skills can be learned by training and experience, most problems arise when professionals are confronted with patients who are depressed because of the course of their disease, and/or when death becomes an impending threat. In this situation, there is a great temptation either to create unrealistic hopes or to pressure patients to 'think positively' in order to 'fight' the cancer. The efficacy of such approaches in terms of cure or extension of life are unproven, although it seems that some patients do feel better when they are able 'to think positively' (De Raeve 1997, p. 250). It must be realized, however, that such an approach might generate two important consequences. First, negative feelings might be marginalized or simply denied, and, second, when faced with a failure to recover, patients may interpret this as a moral failure, i.e. they did not try hard enough (De Raeve 1997, p. 253). It must also be realized that in most cases it is largely an illusion to believe that it is possible to pressure someone to 'find a meaning in the remaining life'. Only they can do this. An outsider can try to help a person contain their anguish, rage or despair in the hope that they will then be able to find their way forwards. This means that the only rule for nurses is to learn to approach patients empathically, to accompany them as an 'understanding friend', being mainly a compassionate listener. It should also not be forgotten that a lively imaginative environment might help patients in overcoming negative phases (De Raeve 1997). Nurses should also encourage patients to undertake everything that might be helpful; for some people this might be a discussion with a psycho-oncologist or a priest, or alternatively participation in social, behavioural or artistic activities.

Quality of life

The second item we wish to raise is quality of life (QoL), including life-maintaining measures. QoL is obviously a relative concept, some aspects of which can clearly be assessed objectively by appropriate means (Slevin et al 1990). Measures of QoL are nowadays used widely in phase III trials in order to determine the place of new cancer treatments in clinical practice, and have contributed to decisions about the utility and efficacy of different therapies (Slevin et al 1990). Nurses should be aware of such results in order to ensure optimal information for patients with cancer. Since most treatments in oncology still remain of a palliative nature, patients have very often to consider the trade-off between the possible utility of treatment and the related probability of an impairment to QoL. Of course, this trade-off is very different when the toxicity of treatment is minimal (e.g. adjuvant therapy with tamoxifen in breast cancer) compared with a toxic chemotherapeutic regimen proposed in the case of advanced non-small cell lung cancer. In the latter case (and in similar clinical situations) nurses should make sure that patients are not simply told that 'there is no other way than to accept this standard treatment'. Such considerations are, of course, the more pertinent the more advanced the disease and the smaller the probability that treatment might prolong survival and/or improve disease-related symptoms.

There is probably no other situation that creates more disagreements within the multiprofessional team than when physicians continue to pressure patients with advanced disease to accept further treatments, while nurses are convinced that this would probably only be detrimental to the QoL of patients. There is only one possible way out of this ethical dilemma: to accept the wishes of the patient, who should of course be adequately informed. Different studies have in fact demonstrated that in such situations the expectations and wishes of staff members may diverge profoundly from those of patients (Slevin et al 1990). This consideration leads us to recognize that there is obviously another, more subjective, meaning associated with QoL, which cannot be assessed objectively: this is the patient's own appreciation of whether or not life is still worth living. First of all, society at large, and health professionals in particular, have to acknowledge death as an inescapable human reality which should not always be postponed by medical treatment. It might be that the core of the resistance to ending life-maintaining measures is a denial of mortality and at the limits of medicine. We should also bear in mind that the dying patient is still a moral actor, and not only a passive victim of disease.

Euthanasia

This discussion leads directly to consideration of one of the ethical dilemmas that currently elicits most controversy, both within society at large and particularly amongst health professionals: euthanasia. The discussion cannot be closed simply by citing the oath of Hippocrates, which is purported to condemn all actions against life. Why should we allow our present decisions to be influenced by someone, however venerable, who lived 2500 years ago, in an entirely different culture (Dupuis 1993)? The debate about euthanasia is profoundly entrenched within the social–cultural reality of each country. Answers to this ethical dilemma might therefore vary in time and according to the prevailing ethical values of a particular society. It should, however, be acknowledged that at least the more developed societies are becoming increasingly pluralistic and therefore that attitudes towards euthanasia might vary according to personal beliefs. This is the principle that has led some countries (e.g. the Netherlands) to decide not to prosecute physicians who carry out active euthanasia (if precise criteria are met) (Dupuis 1993, p. 447), considering that in this situation it is the patient who judges their own life while no value judgements are made about others or about the values of society.

But what about the principle of non-maleficence (do no harm)? According to most ethicists, the duty to do no harm is even stronger than the duty of 'beneficence' (Dupuis 1993, p. 458). However, the duty to do no harm is not inconsistent with active euthanasia in the case of the patient who requests it. We recognize that there is no one attitude that nurses need to take concerning this ethical dilemma. We consider only that it is of paramount importance within each community that this problem be discussed in depth and that the patient remains the focus of attention in any decision-making process. The experience in the Netherlands has shown that such a discussion leads to an important change in the patient–doctor relationship. Patients and doctors (and health professionals in general) tend more and more to make decisions together regarding treatment and its conclusion (Dupuis 1993).

Rationing of healthcare resources

The ethical dilemma of rationing healthcare resources will form our third point for discussion. We will limit ourselves to only a few observations since this topic is mainly of a political nature and it will therefore be considered in Chapter 9, which discusses the political scope of cancer nursing. Both in Europe and in North America, healthcare resources are currently under the combined pressure of raising costs and decreasing resources, whereby the latter is largely determined by political choices favouring the decreasing role of government and an increasing role for market-oriented policies. This situation is bound to have profound consequences for cancer care, since cancer has never been a top priority in the political arena. In the UK, for example, the total expense incurred in relation to the purchase of cyto-toxic drugs is equivalent to the expenditure for only one drug, omeprazole, used in the management of ulcers (B Leonard, personal communication, 1998).

Health professionals, including nurses, should therefore do whatever they can to use available resources in cancer care in the most appropriate way. Costly treatment of unproven value should be avoided, whilst therapies should be limited to treatments derived from evidence-based medicine. However, since many treatments in oncology remain investigational, great care should be taken not to impede further research. Nurses and all health professionals should therefore fight for increasing the research budgets of governments. Moreover, pharmaceutical companies should be obliged to take over a much bigger share of cost of clinical research. The experience of AIDS-militant groups has shown that active engagement of patients and health professionals might influence societal choices. Nurses should therefore become more active in promoting pressure groups led by patients. The experience with breast cancer in the USA has demonstrated that in doing so more resources might be made available for cancer care and research.

RIGHTS OF PATIENTS WITH REGARD TO INFORMATION

The issue of information-giving will now be considered with a particular focus on the often problematic area of informed consent and phase I studies. It is recognized that currently in many countries the question is no longer whether the truth has to be told or not, but rather when, how and through whom the information should be given (Butow et al 1995). However, since ethical attitudes are intimately linked with culture and societal behaviour, there are still instances where health professionals are reluctant to endorse an open policy of information-giving or limit their acceptance to a pure lip-service. Of course, this might not be due in the first instance to a lack of will or to poor training of health professionals, but rather to the overwhelming pressure of society in general, and of families in particular.

In the last 2 years one of the authors (Y.W.-C.) has cared for two young patients (one from southern Italy, the other from the Middle East), whose families demanded that we misinform the patient regarding the goal of cytotoxic treatment. These families requested that the two young female patients should be informed that the only goal of treatment was to allow them to become pregnant later on. Nevertheless, in the end we were able to give more or less correct information.

But would the same result have been achieved if the patients had been treated in their country of origin? Here the societal–cultural pressure would have been quite different, leading perhaps to a rather different result. In these times of rapid globalization it is, however, possible that the sociological background will change more rapidly than one expects. We feel, therefore, that it is important to understand correctly the 'pros and cons' of informing patients with cancer about their illness and treatment, so providing a rational base for either improving the currently used information-giving procedures or, if necessary, developing such procedures. The following sections of this chapter will deal more specifically with the information-giving process, with particular attention to the case of experimental treatments.

Informing patients with cancer

For many centuries physicians managed to avoid telling the truth to patients (Editorial 1996). Ideologically, this was generally justified by means of the Hippocratic oath, which requested that physicians benefit patients and not cause them any harm. Whether this was a genuine reason, or whether physicians found in it a good excuse for avoiding the unpleasant role of the bearer of bad news, is difficult to establish. It must, however, be remembered that physicians' training is centred, to a large extent, on their capacity 'to cure': just giving bad news and recognizing that 'no cure is possible' is something for which clinicians have rarely been trained, at least until recently (A Surbone, personal communication, 1992).

In the past, physicians often also presumed that patients did not really want to know (Editorial 1996). Nowadays, there is little doubt that most patients do want to know their diagnosis, and generally also desire to have a realistic estimation of the prognosis and an exact knowledge of the treatment and its side-effects (Meredith et al 1996). Different studies have also shown that healthcare providers tend to overestimate the possible depressing effect for patients of such information (Cassileth et al 1980, Slevin et al 1990). Patients are generally able to maintain hope and are generally more hopeful, despite having received correct information. They tend also to have a more open attitude towards cancer treatments than people who do not have cancer, including medical and nursing professionals (Slevin et al 1990). We should recognize that protecting patients from the truth may be counter-productive: lack of information can increase uncertainty, anxiety and distress. There is evidence that the level of psychological distress suffered by patients with serious illness is less when they think that they have received adequate information (Kodish, Singer & Siegler 1997).

Since healthcare providers are increasingly recognizing this reality, attitudes and practices have changed markedly during recent decades. This has been particularly true in the USA. For example, Oken in 1961 reported that 90% of physicians did not tell patients the truth about a diagnosis of cancer. This study was repeated 18 years later at the same Chicago hospital, and findings indicated a major shift in physicians' attitudes and practices. In this latter study, 97% of physicians indicated a preference for telling a patient of the diagnosis of cancer (Novack et al 1979).

Research from Europe has demonstrated significant variability in the attitudes of physicians to telling the truth to patients with cancer. Doctors in southern and eastern Europe are more likely to conceal the diagnosis than their counterparts in northern Europe, where the pattern is more similar to that in the USA – even if there are often differences in 'how' the information is provided. There can, however, be little doubt that most patients wish doctors to respect their views rather than those of their family (Benson & Britten 1996). In a study carried out in the UK, which tried to discover patients' views about disclosure of information to their family, results show quite clearly that patients consider that their own needs should take priority over those of their family (Benson & Britten 1996).

Meanwhile, as stated above, ethical choices are never made outside social and political contexts. This means that the results of this latter study may have been different in another cultural or social context. Moreover, we have to take into account that, in most societies, families continue to play a crucial and pivotal role in the whole course of a neoplastic disease. This means that most patients with cancer will be looking for material, psychological and moral support within their familial structure, and that many of them will be unable to deal with the burden of cancer in the absence of such support. In some situations (e.g. terminal care at home) treatment will require the presence of a functioning familial support. Without this, there might be no alternative to hospitalization, as the hospice alternative is available in only a limited number of countries. In practice, it will therefore be important that healthcare providers, while respecting completely the autonomy of patients, attempt to get families involved appropriately in the information and decision-taking process. This is one of the many reasons why patient information-giving always requires a sensitive and empathic attitude on the part of the healthcare provider.

Informing with empathy

Of course, being told the truth without regard to your own wishes can be just as upsetting as being lied to. We must avoid replacing centuries of systematic deception by a new routine of systematic insensitive truth-telling. The majority of healthcare providers have not been taught to break bad news sensitively and supportively (Buckman & Kason 1993). This is where attention to the issues of role enactment and moral strategy, alluded to above, are vitally important.

We must first of all remember that, as in every frightening situation, denial plays an important role in the behaviour of patients with cancer (Butow et al 1995). Denial represents the natural defence against being overburdened with unbearable thoughts when people are unable to cope with them (Gillon 1985). Denial is a basic psychological mechanism that health providers have to take seriously into account when they are planning disclosure of bad news to patients.

It must be remembered that patients also have the right not to know, and it is advisable to let the patient decide when information should be given. Through sensitive questioning or through offering various possibilities to ask questions, physicians and nurses should generally be able to understand when the best moment to provide information has come. Then the patient should not be compelled to wait 'till someone has time to speak', but has the right to receive the information from one health professional who is trusted. It is also important to realize that information-giving is not something 'which is done once for ever', but that it is rather a continuous and delicate process. Information needs to be repeated, to be rephrased, to be adapted to the knowledge and cultural background of the patient. It happens rather often that during the first conversation the patient will pick up only parts of the information given; over the following days the denial process can also erase the most unpleasant components of the truth (Tomamichel et al 1995). This is the very background that leads to a situation we often encounter in our clinical areas: the nurse feels that the information given by the physician has been 'partial or wrong', while the latter is convinced that everything important has been said. Therefore, one of the most important duties in cancer care is to promote continued discussion between medical and nursing staff about the degree of information given to patients.

Some of the principles discussed below concerning informing patients eligible for experimental treatments might prove useful also in the general process of information-giving. Next to learning when the information procedure has to be started, we also need to learn how to support and assist patients as they absorb and understand the nature of their medical situation. Empathy remains a cornerstone of the necessary attitude of healthcare providers. Modern information procedures strive to respect the autonomy of patients; however, this autonomy can be real and realistic only if the patient is not overburdened with all kinds of problems. For example, if the patient is depressed, if he or she does not have the necessary support of a family or partner, or if the social situation is disastrous, we might imagine many factors that might so overwhelm a patient that autonomy and respect might not mean much more than an ideological slogan. Our empathy and our engagement should be directed towards reducing the social, psychological and human burden of the patients, so that they can function autonomously. This, of course, cannot be the sole task of the nurse, but is something that can be dealt with only by the whole caring team, including psychologists and social workers.

Thus it is possible to summarize key points in the information process:

- Not only the quality of the information, but also the quality of the informing person, is essential.
- Information has to be individualized.
- Language must be understandable.

- A nurse should be present when a physician is informing.
- The information process should take place as a part of the collaboration between physician and nurse.
- Staff must be informed about the information that has been imparted.
- Last, but not least, information-giving is a continuous process.

Information procedures for experimental treatments

The distinction between evidence-based or standardized treatments and experimental approaches is anything but sharp. The continuous introduction of new regimens and novel drugs prompts a situation in which only a very few cancer treatments can be regarded as being definitely 'state of the art'. Because of this, some authors (Tattersall et al 1994) have requested that the information given to most patients treated with chemotherapy should be very similar to that which is requested for those who are asked to enter an experimental protocol. While this question remains currently controversial, a better knowledge about how we should proceed to inform patients who are considered to be eligible for experimental trials may improve our overall ability correctly to inform all patients with cancer. This requires, however, that we briefly discuss the ethical base of experimental studies.

The Nuremberg Code and the Helsinki Declaration

The Nuremberg Code is the most important document in the history of the ethics of medical research (Shuster 1997). The code was formulated in August 1947 at the end of the judgement of Nazi doctors accused of conducting murderous and torturous human experiments in the concentration camps. It served as a blueprint for today's principles that ensure the rights of subjects in medical research. The judges at Nuremberg recognized that more was necessary to protect human research subjects than the maxim *primum non nocere* and Hippocratic ethics. Accordingly, they articulated a set of 10 principles centred not on the physician but on the research subject (Grodin & Annas 1996). These principles, which are now known as the Nuremberg Code, included among others the absolute requirement of informed consent and the right of the subject to withdraw from participation in an experiment.

In the traditional Hippocratic doctor–patient relationship, once patients agree to be treated, they are viewed as totally compliant to the beneficent and trusted physician. In research, which may be outside the beneficent context of the physician–patient relationship, the situation is different, because the physician's primary goal is to test a scientific hypothesis by following protocol. The key contribution of Nuremberg was to merge Hippocratic ethics and the protection of human rights into a single code. This not only required that researchers protect the best interest of their subjects but also proclaimed that subjects can actively protect themselves as well. The Nuremberg Code profoundly influenced the various versions of the Declaration of Helsinki promulgated by the World Medical Association since 1964 which, furthermore, established the necessity for peer review of scientific research and therefore set the basis for establishing institutional ethics committees (Council for International Organizations of Medical Sciences 1993).

Phase I studies as a paradigmatic example

Phase I studies are a paradigmatic example (the reason why they are discussed rather than phase II or III studies) of the difficult ethical problems involved in therapeutic cancer research and are, therefore, of pivotal importance in terms of information-giving procedures. The main goal of phase I studies is to assess the toxicity of a new drug and to determine the maximum tolerated dose and the dose to be recommended for subsequent disease-oriented phase II studies.

There are many ethical issues related to the conduct of phase I studies. Some of these relate to the treatment of patients at ineffective or toxic doses, low probability of response, unknown toxic effects and benefits of the new agent, difficulty of obtaining adequate informed consent in vulnerable patients, and discrepancy between the objectives of the investigators and those of the patients. In fact, while the overall response rate in these studies is lower than 5% (Decoster, Stein & Holdener 1990), patients with cancer who participate are strongly motivated by the hope of therapeutic benefit (Sessa & Cavalli 1990). Altruistic feelings appear to have a limited role in motivating patients to participate in these trials. A recent study also demonstrated that, while patients appear to have an adequate self-perceived knowledge of the risk of investigational agents, only a minority of them appear to understand fully the purpose of phase I trials as dose-determination studies (Daugherty et al 1995). This is possibly because such recognition would decrease a patient's hope of a therapeutic result. It is therefore understandable that these patients are particularly vulnerable to biased or ill-conceived information.

The problem of informed consent is even more compelling, and involves more ethical and legal challenges, when children are involved.

Optimizing information

In order to render information procedures more explicit, we briefly describe here the experience of one of the authors (Y.W.-C.) over the past 10 years. First, it is of paramount importance to test among healthcare staff acquainted with each patient the possibility of offering a phase I drug, taking into account medical, social and psychological aspects. If the patient is deemed to be eligible, we adopt an information procedure (Willems & Sessa 1989) based on a modified version of the approach proposed by Rodenhuis et al (1984). During an initial conversation the patient is informed by the treating physician of the possibility of receiving an experimental treatment. If the patient shows interest, a second appointment is scheduled for approximately 1 week hence. This appointment should include the patient, the patient's relatives or friends, the physician responsible for the experimental study and the research nurse. At this stage at least the following essential information should be conveyed to the patient:

- The lack of other treatments of greater efficacy
- That the experimental drug has so far been evaluated in animals but, if at all, only in a few humans
- That the antitumour effect is not only unknown but probably unlikely
- That there is only limited knowledge about possible side-effects
- That participation in the study implies more frequent hospital visits
- That the patient has the option of withdrawing at any stage, or refusing the treatment without compromising their future medical care.

Further appointments are arranged if these are requested by the patient. Only at the end of this information-giving process will a consent form be signed by the patient, a witness and the physician. In our experience, about two thirds of patients will eventually accept the phase I drug and most of them will recall the essential information even after several months (Willems & Sessa 1989).

In a more recent study we tried to assess the three dimensions of the information-giving process: the information itself, the emotional aspect and the interactive aspects (Tomamichel et al 1995). Although the overall information-giving procedure was evaluated as being both positive and comprehensive, even experienced physicians were still found to have problems with the interactive dimension. Unsatisfactory results were in fact reported on the items related to the doctor's awareness of the indirect expressed anxieties and messages of the patients. These conclusions highlight the fact that there is probably no 'definite answer' to the question of how best to inform patients in experimental trials. This is an ongoing and continuous process, and we consider therefore that each institution actively engaged in experimental studies should also be involved in studies investigating the information-giving process employed by staff. These studies will serve as a necessary quality control of the information given to patients.

The present discussion should have clarified that optimal information is an ethical prerequisite for experimental studies in oncology. Since most cancer treatments still remain investigational, this experience should also form the basis for optimizing the information given to most patients with cancer. The various health professionals (doctors, nurses, social workers, etc.) have hereby a different role, which may vary according to the organizational scheme of each institution. Specific implications for the role of the nurses in daily practice are discussed in other chapters of this book.

CONCLUSION

Consideration of ethical issues in healthcare practice raises our awareness of some of the most fundamental questions surrounding human interaction, issues, for example, concerning the appropriate balance between respect for persons and individual autonomy, and the beneficent paternalism that is not only enshrined in healthcare provision, but also mirrored in normal human social existence. Families and communities provide support and nurture for those who are vulnerable and in need. In healthcare, and arguably particularly in care of patients suffering from cancer, patients can have many needs and most are vulnerable. How do we effectively and ethically meet their needs while fully respecting the human being who is our patient? We have argued in this chapter that we need to begin by examining and exploring some of our basic assumptions, assumptions that we hold regarding both our patients and our practice. Examples of some of these assumptions have been drawn out under the heading 'Incidents from practice' pages 161 to 163 in this chapter. We have also suggested that the issue of information-giving, particularly information-giving before a patient consents to participate in a phase I study, may provide us with valuable insight into both respecting and protecting our patients.

As we move into the next century, great challenges face us in terms of healthcare provision and practice. The rapid changes in care and the unprecedented number of new and experimental treatments for cancer sufferers show little sign of abating. This perpetuates the difficulties already discussed above regarding appropriate information-giving to patients. However, other issues, briefly mentioned above, are also likely to focus the attention of both the practitioner and the cancer sufferer as we move into the new millennium. These are issues such as that regarding the ethical appropriateness of treating patients with either ineffective or toxic doses of drugs, or using drugs with low probability of response or unknown toxic effects. There is also the ever-present difficulty of obtaining adequate consent in ill, vulnerable patients. This is exacerbated by the potentially divergent perceptions and objectives between patient and practitioner or researcher. These are just some of the ethical problems and dilemmas that we currently carry with us into, and which are likely to become pressing issues in, this century. This is, of course, only a small element of the ethical problems facing patients and researchers and practitioners who investigate or try to treat their cancers and care for them as human beings. Stem cell transplantation, genetic screening and gene therapy are other equally problematic areas of concern. Perhaps the Aristotelian concern with the character-istics of the virtuous person was never of greater importance as we try to equip the practitioner and researcher to work humanely with patients with cancer in the twenty-first century.

REFERENCES

Aristotle 1980 The nicomachean ethics, translated by Sir David Ross, revised by J L Ackrill & J O Urmson. Oxford University Press, Oxford

Bandeman E L, Bandeman B 1995 Nursing ethics through the life span, 3rd edn. Prentice Hall International, Englewood Cliffs, New Jersey

Beauchamps T L, Childress J F 1989 Principles of biomedical ethics, 3rd edn. Oxford University Press, Oxford

Benson J, Britten N 1996 Respecting the autonomy of cancer patients when talking with their families: qualitative analysis of semi-structured interviews with patients. British Medical Journal 313:729–731

Bok S 1984 Secrets: on the ethics of concealment and revelation. Oxford University Press, Oxford

Buckman R, Kason Y 1993 How to break bad news – a practical guide for healthcare professionals. Macmillan, London

Butow P N, Dunn S M, Tattersall M H N 1995 Communication with cancer patients: does it matter? Journal of Palliative Care 11:34–38

Carr-Hill R, Dixon P 1992 Skill mix in the effectiveness of nursing care. York Centre for Health Economics, University of York, York

Cassileth B R, Zupkis R V, Sutton-Smith K, March V 1980 Information and participation preferences among cancer patients. Annals of Internal Medicine 92(6):832–836

Council for International Organizations of Medical Sciences 1993 International ethical guidelines for biomedical research involving human subjects. Council for International Organizations of Medical Sciences, Geneva

Daugherty C, Ratain M J, Grochowski E, Stocking C, Kodish E, Mick R, Siegler M 1995 Perceptions of cancer patients and their physicians involved in phase I trials. Journal of Clinical Oncology 13(5):1062–1072

Decoster G, Stein G, Holdener E E 1990 Responses and toxic death in phase I clinical trials. Annals of Oncology 1:171–174

De Raeve L 1997 Positive thinking and moral oppression in cancer care. European Journal of Cancer Care 6:248–256

Downie R S 1964 Government, action and morality. MacMillan, London

Downie R S, Calman K 1996 Healthy respect, 2nd edn. Oxford University Press, Oxford

DuBois E R, Hamel R, O'Connell L J (eds) 1994 A matter of principles? Ferment in US bioethics. Trinity Press International, Valley Forge, Pennsylvania

Dupuis H M 1993 Euthanasia in the Netherlands: facts and moral arguments. Annals of Oncology 4:447–450

Editorial 1996 Talking to patients about cancer. No excuse now for not doing it. British Medical Journal 313:699–700

Edwards S D 1996 Nursing ethics: a principle-based approach. MacMillan, Basingstoke, UK

Ford P, Walsh M 1994 New rituals for old: nursing through the looking glass. Butterworth–Heinemann, Oxford

Gillon R 1985 Telling the truth and medical ethics. British Medical Journal 291:1556–1557

Grodin M A, Annas G J 1996 Legacies of Nuremberg: medical ethics and human rights. Journal of the American Medical Association 276:1682–1683

Hospers J 1961 An introduction to philosophical analysis. Routledge & Kegan Paul, London

Kant I 1991 The metaphysics of morals, translated by Mary Gregor. Cambridge University Press, Cambridge

Kodish E, Singer P A, Siegler M 1997 Ethical issues. In: De Vita V T, Hellman S, Rosenberg S A (eds) Cancer: principles and practice of oncology, 5th edn. Lippincott–Raven, Philadelphia, PA, p 2973

Levine M E 1977 Nursing ethics and the ethical nurse. American Journal of Nursing 77(5):845–849

Lundt B, Neale C 1987 A comparison of hospice and hospital: care goals set by staff. Palliative Medicine 1:136–148

Meredith C, Symonds P, Webster L, Lamont D, Pyper E, Gillis C R, Fallowfield L 1996 Information needs of cancer patients in west Scotland: cross sectional survey of patients' views. British Medical Journal 313:724–726

Mill J S 1993 Utilitarianism, on liberty, considerations on representative government, 3rd edn. Everyman Library, London

Morse J 1991 Negotiating commitment and involvement in the nurse–patient relationship. Journal of Advanced Nursing 16:455–468

Morse J M, Doberneck B 1995 Delineating the concept of hope. Image: Journal of Nursing Scholarship 274:275–285

Novack D H, Plumer R, Smith R L, Ochitill H, Morrow G R, Bennett J M 1979 Changes in physicians, attitudes towards the cancer patient. Journal of the American Medical Association 241(9):897–900

Oken D 1961 What to tell cancer patients: a study of medical attitudes. Journal of the American Medical Association 175:1120–1123

Randall F, Downie R S 1996 Palliative care ethics: a good companion. Oxford University Press, Oxford

Rodenhuis S, Van den Heuvel W J, Annyas A A, Koops H S, Sleijfer D T, Mulder N H 1984 Patient motivation and informed consent in phase I study of an anticancer agent. European Journal of Cancer and Clinical Oncology 20(4):457–462

Rumbold G 1986 Ethics in nursing practice. Baillière Tindall, Eastbourne, UK

Scott P A 1993 Virtue, moral imagination and the health care practitioner. PhD thesis, University of Glasgow, Glasgow

Scott P A 1995a Aristotle, nursing and health care ethics. Nursing Ethics 2(4):279–285

Scott P A 1995b Care, attention and imaginative identification in nursing practice. Journal of Advanced Nursing 21:1196–1200

Scott P A 1995c Role, role enactment and the health care practitioner. Journal of Advanced Nursing 22:323–328

Scott P A 1997 Imagination in practice. Journal of Medical Ethics 23:45–50

Scott P A 1998 Professional ethics: are we on the wrong track? Nursing Ethics 5(6):477–485

Scott P A 1999 Autonomy, power and control in palliative care. Cambridge Quarterly of Health Care Ethics 8(2):139–147

Seale C 1989 What happens in hospices: a review of the research evidence. Social Science and Medicine 28(6):551–559

Sessa C, Cavalli F 1990 Who benefits from phase I studies? Annals of Oncology 1:164–165 (editorial)

Shuster E 1997 Fifty years later: the significance of the Nuremberg Code. New England Journal of Medicine 337:1436–1440

Slevin M L, Stubbs L, Plant H J, Wilson P, Gregory W M, Armes P J, Downer S M 1990 Attitudes to chemotherapy: comparing views of patients with cancer with those of doctors, nurses, and general public. British Medical Journal 300(6737):1458–1460

Smart J J C 1973 An outline of a system of utilitarian ethics. In: Smart J J C, Williams B (eds) Utilitarianism: for and against. Cambridge University Press, Cambridge, p 3

Tattersall M H N, Butow P N, Griffin A M, Dunn S M 1994 The take-home message: patients prefer consultation audiotapes to summary letters. Journal of Clinical Oncology 12:1305–1311

Tomamichel M, Sessa C, Herzig S, De Jong J, Pagani O, Willems Y, Cavalli F 1995 Informed consent for phase I studies: evaluation of quantity and quality of information provided to patients. Annals of Oncology 6:363–369

Willems Y, Sessa C 1989 Informing patients about phase I trials. How should it be done? Acta Oncologica 28:106–107

Towards a European framework for cancer nursing services

Alison Ferguson   Nora Kearney

CHAPTER 9

INTRODUCTION

From an examination of the material presented in the preceding chapters of this book spring common themes. The authors will draw upon these themes in constructing a developmental framework for advancing cancer nursing. This is done against a backdrop of professional diversity and political change in Europe. Nevertheless, the authors wish to put forward a framework that builds on existing strengths in partnerships and collaborative working to expand and fulfil the potential of cancer nurses across Europe.

In our daily lives, local work pressures can crowd out the desire to look outwards and observe what is going on elsewhere. Yet, as the world appears to turn faster and to shrink in size, the opportunities to learn from events and issues outside our immediate experience become greater. For example, close involvement by the authors in recent years in shaping cancer nursing services within England and Scotland has afforded the opportunity to consider the wider context of cancer care, commissioning services that meet patient and user needs within many cultural perspectives as well as coordinating the multiple factors inherent in the delivery of cancer services. Involvement at a national, as well as a European, level has required the authors to adopt a strategic approach to the development of cancer nursing services which has its roots in clinical care and professional development. The ideas presented in this chapter draw upon these experiences.

In this chapter we would like to consider the recent developments in cancer nursing (some of which are presented earlier in this text) and, building on new information, propose a dynamic structure that will support the development of cancer nurses for the new millennium. First, because cancer nursing does not operate in a vacuum and is responsive to the needs of the public as a whole, we will consider current political, social and health trends and perspectives (readers should be especially mindful of the timing of this book and in particular the very difficult situation being faced by nurses where conflict remains an integral part of everyday life). Second, we will review the history of both cancer nursing and nursing generally from a European perspective. Finally, we will propose a framework appropriate to the challenges of the future – a framework that will encourage progress within cancer nursing care that is sensitive and supportive of the multicultural context of Europe.

THE EUROPEAN CONTEXT

Europe is a loose geographical definition encompassing many cultures and languages. Following the Second World War the European map was redrawn and remained fairly stable until the late 1980s, when unprecedented changes took place in Central and Eastern Europe, and the former USSR became the Newly Independent States. Thus, while Europe was composed of 32 Member States in the early 1980s, this has risen to more than 50 during the 1990s, and current unrest in the Balkans suggests that the final map of Europe may remain fluid for many years to come.

The changes that have taken place in Central and Eastern Europe and the Newly Independent States have been accompanied by severe social and economic difficulties, and at times military conflict. Such changes have a continuing and as yet immeasurable impact on the rest of Europe. They have contributed to an increasing divide between Eastern and Western states.

Added to this, increased public expectations in Western states for improved healthcare exaggerates the mismatch with ever decreasing resources. In Europe, as in other developed nations of the world, other contributing factors to healthcare include: the changing demographics of our society, particularly an increasingly aged population; increasing population mobility throughout Europe; the emergence of new diseases and the reappearance of old communicable diseases coupled with costly technological developments resulting from new scientific knowledge. Nursing is not immune to these pressures and, indeed, in a number of European countries nurses find themselves central to such changes as it is nurses who are often seen as providing answers to the shortfall in government spending.

COMMON THEMES FROM THE LATE TWENTIETH CENTURY TO THE TWENTY-FIRST CENTURY

The issues outlined above are considered below in more detail. Common themes from the end of the twentieth century in terms of population demographics, lifestyles, patterns of disease, treatment, research advances and public opinion give some indication as to how the future may look through the twenty-first century. It is important to distinguish, where possible, between Western European attitudes and trends, which are often dominant, with the customs, desires and aspirations of the Eastern European countries, about which we are generally less familiar. For this reason we have labelled trends 'Western' or 'Eastern' to distinguish between the primary direction of influence.

Demographic time bomb

The demographic time bomb has been discussed and debated increasingly. The population of around 850 million is expected to increase slowly. Fertility rates are falling, as are marriages, while divorce is on the increase. The number of 60–79-year-olds is increasing, while the economically active population is decreasing (Ludvigsen & Roberts 1996). In other words, there are increasingly fewer people of working age supporting those who require greater input in terms of health and social care.

Lifestyles and culture

Cultural, social, political and economic factors between Eastern and Western states are currently diverse. However, there are already examples of Eastern block countries aspiring to the products and services available to Western populations. Increasingly, similarities may spread as has happened among Western European countries (European Union Publication (EUP) 1997a,b). Languages may be shared and a common language of Europe may emerge.

Patterns of disease: return to public health

The increasing demands upon healthcare together with a resurgence of old communicable diseases has focused the minds of East and West upon the value of health and social prevention of disease and health and social promotion. Nurses have always played an important role in this arena and will continue to do so in the future (Salvage & Heijnen 1997).

Treatment and research advances: technological innovation

Technological advances and innovations in communication will impact upon all industries and services, influencing the speed and accuracy with which information can be transferred between individuals, organizations, services and countries. The huge gap in access to technology between the Western and Eastern European countries will reduce. The crisis facing Eastern European countries due to their neglect of the healthcare system is mirrored by the unprecedented demand made by Western Europeans upon their already overstretched services.

Lucrative technical product developments by multi-million dollar drug and treatment companies may enable the Eastern expansion of existing products currently available in the West. Such companies will be able to utilize technologies in developing innovative and interactive education mediums for professionals, patients and carers within Europe and worldwide.

Novel information technology equipment will be used in the twenty-first century to record and process patient data in far greater detail than is possible today. Outcome, in terms of quality of life, mortality and treatment history, will all be recorded electronically and processed to predict treatment and care required, so that resources can be allocated with far greater accuracy. However, it should be remembered that whilst technological advances may contain costs they will also have cost implications.

The cost–quality–service connection

For the future, concerns around cost effectiveness that have strengthened in the 1990s will continue to gather momentum. Developments in the USA have led to concern for close links between costs and service delivery. Such a relationship has manifested itself in the development of patient care processes such as diagnostic related groups (DRGs). The greater influence of insurance companies upon treatment and care decisions has resulted in considerably more paperwork for clinicians. Delegation of cost concerns to the service user and payment for service at the point of delivery has heralded a whole new emphasis upon responsibility and accountability. It has also fuelled an increased interest among service users to exercise their right to have a greater say in services provided.

Public opinion, awareness and involvement

In Western Europe there has been an increasing awareness by the population at large in their health and an increasing desire for information and responsibility. Such demands upon healthcare professionals will continue to challenge their desire to marry up patient partnership and the provision of evidence-based treatment and care. As costs increase and governments and individuals find it more difficult to support healthcare requirements, the public, in the form of charities and the voluntary sector, are likely to play an increasing role. Eastern European countries have always relied heavily on the contribution of the extended family in healthcare. This type of model may suggest affordable alternatives to Western States.

Attention to quality standards, benchmarks, quality in terms of patient care and staff development, recruitment and retention

The Western European countries have seen the drive to improve quality and to cut costs. Such a drive for efficiency, together with increasing public involvement in health service provision, has led to the desire to meet set standards and to compare practices through objective measures. In this way, high-quality care can be identified and supported.

Key social and health trends and their resulting impact on cancer treatment and care are summarized in Boxes 9.1 and 9.2. Such trends, also noted by Corner (1991), are predicted to continue as core themes influencing the development of cancer services for the new millennium.

> ■ BOX 9.1 Predicated European health changes impacting on cancer treatment and care
>
> 1. Increased burden on services due to elderly population
> 2. Public involvement and responsibility for health
> 3. Focus upon health promotion and disease prevention
> 4. Specialization of health services
> 5. Standardization and bench-marking of services

> ■ BOX 9.2 Current and future trends in cancer services
>
> 1. Specialization of medical and nursing services
> 2. Integration of palliative care acroos all care areas and earlier in treatment
> 3. Increased consumer choice
> 4. Cancer education for primary care professionals

COLLABORATIVE APPROACHES IN EUROPE

The European Commission produces an annual programme of work for the year ahead. In the early 1990s the focus of activity centred upon legislation in joining the western and central countries in legal and monetary union, and agreeing joint protocols in terms of social and employment rights. Since the Treaty of Maastricht in 1993 the mid and late 1990s have seen a prevalence of consultation documents for future policy and action including possible legislation on employment conditions, discussions on minimum wage and on equal opportunities for disabled people (EUP 1997a,b). There have also been a number of proposals for new EU public health arrangements relating to pollution and related diseases, rare diseases, and accidents and injuries. From such initiatives, templates for collaborative work in healthcare have been set.

For example, in November 1993 the European Commission published its response to the new health provisions in the Treaty of Maastricht. Its Communication on the framework for action in the field of public health identified the following areas for future community action (Ludvigsen & Roberts 1996):

1. Health promotion, education and training

2. Health data and indicators, and monitoring and surveillance of diseases

3. Cancer

4. Drugs

5. Acquired immune deficiency syndrome and other communicable diseases

6. Intentional and unintentional accidents and injuries

7. Pollution-related diseases

8. Rare diseases

Some have argued that public health action cannot be fully understood by means of the Commission's disease-by-disease approach alone. Instead the specific circumstances of various disease categories must be considered: age groups, vulnerable groups and specific environments. Such an interdisciplinary, horizontal approach is consistent with the skills and perspectives demonstrated by trained cancer nurses. Thus, the opportunities for cancer nurses in leading service and clinical developments – and ultimately patient outcomes – are immense.

There already are many examples of collaborative cancer initiatives taking place across Europe. In the late 1980s and 1990s the European Commission funded research projects into cancer treatment, care and education, and through such projects has highlighted the need for joint strategies to fight cancer. Protocols for joint working and collaboration are encouraged. In addition, a large number of educational projects, ranging from 1 or 2 days to over 2 years, has been funded (Bond & Jodrell 1997, Jodrell 1997) (see Chapter 5 for an illustration of these projects). Any future framework for cancer services takes place in the context of these European developments.

NURSING IN EUROPE

Nursing in itself is a formidable force. While exact numbers are not known, there is no doubt that nurses form the largest group of healthcare professionals in Europe and account for between 40% and 60% of healthcare spending. It is estimated that around five million nurses serve a European population of around 850 million (Asvall 1997). Yet, as stated by Asvall, the World Health Organization (WHO) Regional Director for Europe: 'In many, if not most, European countries, these health professionals (nurses) do not get the recognition they deserve, or the working facilities they need to carry out their unique function in our health care systems' (Asvall 1997, p. xiii). This may be attributed to the lack of a common strategy for nurses in Europe and a reflection on the diversity of nursing as a profession across this large geographical region.

Whilst few nurses would disagree with Asvall, there is some evidence that nurses, and the value they bring to society, are recognized in terms of their provision of care. Indeed, nurses have been identified as the most cost-effective resource for delivering high-quality public health and clinical packages (World Bank 1993). It has been claimed that, although nursing does not attract the same attention as issues such as the commercialization of medicine or the emergency supply of drugs, it could arguably have a greater impact on health services (Salvage 1993). Such recognition is a long way from nursing's roots.

THE GROWING PROFESSIONALIZATION OF NURSING

In 1900, nurses were little more than handmaidens to doctors. In the UK, Florence Nightingale had established her school at St Thomas' Hospital in London, yet there was limited recognition that nurses required training to undertake the tasks expected of them. Many writers since have argued that, from the beginning, Florence Nightingale saw nursing as central to the care process of the sick and fundamental in the promotion of wellness.

Throughout this century a number of developments have influenced the perception of nurse preparation and status. The development of specific roles and training, including university preparation, has enabled nurses to offer advanced skills in diagnosis, treatment and care. New specialist roles have helped to raise the profile of a particular disease or the needs of a special client group as well as nurses' profile (Carroll 1998, Corner 1995, Patiraki-Kourbani et al 1998). Since the roles that nurses have traditionally played in education and liaison have become increasingly important to their healthcare colleagues, there has been a greater understanding and merging of responsibilities. Similarly, professions allied to medicine (PAMs) have developed their area of practice, resulting in overlaps with services provided by nurses (Page et al 1998), for example in lymphoedema, radiotherapy and communication (Ferguson et al 1998). The Eastern European countries are far less sophisticated in their development of nurses and nursing. Nevertheless, nurses are recognized for the public health role they play within the healthcare team.

Cancer nursing has been a relatively recent specialist development. It, too, has developed a voice within its own specialty and is beginning to influence healthcare at large. The challenge for the twenty-first century for cancer nurses will be to maximize the impact of expertise available in cancer nursing to related areas of care. It is this area and degree of influence that will change substantially in the twenty-first century.

Throughout this book, differences in cancer nursing across Europe have been alluded to and, from this, strengths and weaknesses can be identified. What seems clear from the evidence presented is that cancer nursing itself is a strong discipline, and indeed is often identified as a model for other specialist groups to replicate.

THE POLITICAL VOICE OF CANCER NURSING

At the close of the twentieth century, cancer nurses have a justifiable reputation for making their opinions known and for finding forums in which they can establish a rapport with their patients, healthcare colleagues and the powerful bodies of countries and governments. A number of influential organizations have been established by cancer nurses. Their pioneering spirit and drive has led to developments in standards for practice, registration and training, and professional development in Europe and America, which other nursing disciplines seek to emulate.

There are a number of organizations that cancer nurses have created in order to strengthen their collective voice. The most notable of these within Europe is the European Oncology Nursing Society (EONS). EONS was developed in 1984 following informal discussions amongst European nurses spearheaded by Robert Tiffany. The Society was established as a federation of oncology nursing societies, institutions and agencies involved in cancer care, and in 1997 individual nurses were also able to become full members of the Society. Currently EONS has a membership of 23 National Oncology Nursing Societies and 207 individual members representing 22 300 nurses in 30 countries. Through a range of activities across Europe, EONS has, in a relatively short space of time, become an important political player in cancer care in Europe. Through collaboration with the European Commission (particularly the Europe Against Cancer Programme), the Advisory Committee for Training in Nursing (ACTN), the Standing Committee of Nurses in the European Union (PCN) and the WHO. EONS has ensured that the voice of cancer nursing is heard at a European level and, as a consequence, the needs of cancer nurses are being addressed.

In addition to this political development, EONS is identified as leading the way in education and practice development issues for nurses in Europe. The development of the EONS core curriculum for a post-basic course in cancer nursing (EONS 1990) heralded similar developments in other areas of nursing. The momentum that EONS has established in terms of raising the profile of cancer nursing will be important to maintain as we begin a new millennium.

It is important to acknowledge, however, that nurses do not deliver cancer care in isolation: optimal care delivery is dependent upon a multiprofessional approach to care. The concept of collaboration is crucial if we are to improve outcomes for patients with cancer. To this end, the alliance that is inherent within the Federation of European Cancer Societies (FECS) is one of EONS' greatest strengths. FECS is composed of the European Association of Cancer Research, European Oncology Nursing Society, European Society of Medical Oncology, European Society of Surgical Oncology, European Society of Therapeutic Radiology and Oncology, and the European branch of the International Society of Paediatric Oncology. The main aim of FECS is to promote and coordinate collaboration between these societies. As a full member of this Federation, EONS ensures nursing is accepted as an equal partner in cancer care, an important message to relay across Europe given the diversity of the status of nursing at a European level.

In developing cancer nursing in Europe, EONS has also developed relationships with the International Society for Nurses in Cancer Care (ISNCC), the Oncology Nursing Society of the USA and the International Union of Cancer Control (Union Internacional Contra la Cancrum; UICC). Such relationships will lead to a comprehensive approach to developing cancer nursing internationally and can only strengthen the voice of cancer nurses.

However, whilst there is no doubt that cancer nursing has progressed over the past decade, there is much that remains to be achieved before we can identify the specialty of cancer nursing Europe-wide. The differences and constraints imposed by diverse levels of technological access, healthcare information and provision suggest that it would be inappropriate to adopt a framework that did not take account of these differences. These points are discussed more fully below.

CANCER NURSING IN EUROPE: SURVEY

The availability of accurate information precludes detailed information of current services in cancer nursing across the whole European region. To provide an overview of cancer nursing in Europe, a small survey was conducted with EONS members in 1996–97, and the results are presented here. Notably not all countries are yet represented (e.g. many of the new countries in Eastern Europe). A questionnaire was sent to one representative nurse member of each country currently represented (Box 9.3). It asked them to describe how cancer care was currently provided and to give their opinion as to how the situation may change in the next millennium. The results from this study provide a snapshot of current similarities and differences across a range of older and more recent Member States.

It should be noted that countries responding to the questionnaire are primarily those that would be considered to have Western buying power and Western healthcare values. There were a range of responses that partly reflected the status of the country in terms of complexity of healthcare provided. Respondents were asked a number of questions related to the delivery of cancer nursing in their country. Responses are grouped and presented under theme headings.

■ BOX 9.3   EONS representation in Europe

	Represented by EONS	Not represented by EONS
Western Europe	Austria Belgium Denmark* Finland France Germany* Greece* Iceland* Ireland* Israel Italy* Malta The Netherlands Norway Portugal Spain Sweden Switzerland* Turkey UK*	
Central and Eastern Europe	Slovenia* Poland	Albania Bulgaria Croatia Czech Republic Slovakia Macedonia Newly independent states
Republics of the former USSR	Estonia*	Armenia Azerbaijan Belarus Georgia Kazakhstan Kyrgyzstan Latvia Lithuania Republic of Moldova The Russian Federation Tajikistan Turkmenistan Ukraine Uzbekistan

*Written response to questionnaire received.

The context of cancer care

Cancer care is provided in a range of healthcare settings, including acute, outpatient clinics, community and rehabilitation settings, and home care. In Switzerland and the UK, statements were made about the move towards providing care on an outpatient basis as much as possible. Estonia, however, provides care in two specified cancer centres: in a small country, this seems to work efficiently.

Qualifications and training for cancer nurses

Nurses in Switzerland, Denmark and the UK have post-basic qualifications in cancer nursing up to PhD level, although only a very few have Master's or PhD qualifications. Cancer nurses receive a range of education from nurse educators, physicians, psychologists (Denmark) and members of the healthcare team, usually within specialist cancer centres and universities in the technologically resourced countries. In Iceland, nurses receive diploma- and degree-level education in cancer care, while all advanced nurses obtain Master's level courses or PhDs from the USA. In Estonia, nurses learn within their workplace. For Estonia the vision for the future is that cancer nursing will be recognized as an independent specialty that requires a university education.

Two or three respondents commented on developments in general education for cancer nurses and how it lacked standardization. Differences in cancer education are complicated by differences in the levels and characteristics of general training in nursing, medicine and healthcare, although there is a trend towards university level education and an abandonment of pre-registration specialization.

Perception by other nurses and the public

The perception of the cancer nurse by other nurses and by the public is positive and fairly similar across respondents. The cancer nurse is respected as undertaking a complex job, considered by the public to be proficient and more qualified than other nurses. Cancer nurses are regarded in Germany and Yugoslavia as an identifiable and cohesive group. In Switzerland, the public may not fully appreciate the subspecialty of cancer nursing, but when they do there is respect – out of awe for the emotionally laden aspect of the work.

The effect of national and European issues
upon cancer care

Respondents said little about the current European issues that affect or may affect their practice. This was surprising considering that these nurses have been motivated enough to join a European society. On the other hand, their unfamiliarity with the issues reflects the general public's lack of clarity around Europe. National issues that might have a more general impact upon healthcare seemed to be of greatest concern; these included cost-cutting and efficiency measures.

Conclusions from the survey

From this limited survey, similarities were identified across Europe. Nurses responding to the survey were generally positive about their chosen discipline and the contribution they were perceived to make to healthcare. However, the views of many countries, particularly the less developed, are not included in the survey. The number of differences in culture and circumstances outlined suggests that seeking a common framework for cancer services and nurse preparation across cancer nurses in Europe may be unrealistic. However, there are certainly common principles and much has been gained to date through sharing the EONS core curriculum, which has provided a common basis for preparation and practice. In addition, the development of a cancer nursing network made possible by the EONS infrastructure facilitates a common approach to advancing cancer nursing practice in Europe.

ADVANCED CANCER NURSING ROLES

Developments in cancer nursing worldwide have led to a plethora of roles identified for cancer nurses. Such diversity of cancer nursing practice has led to confusion both within and outwith the profession, particularly in relation to advanced cancer nursing practice. In a recent review of the literature, Knowles & Kearney (1998) concluded that, at present, there seems to be little consensus as to what constitutes an advanced practitioner in terms of educational or clinical preparation. Despite this, however, nurses have not been slow to embrace the new roles, even though they appear to be driven by economic rather than professional ideals. Such developments in Europe perhaps weaken the position of nurses and make the need for a comprehensive strategy all the more apparent.

In the first action plan of the European Commission's 'Europe Against Cancer' (EAC) programme (1987–1989) it was proposed that 'every Member State should recognise the specialist nature of oncology' and take action relating to the training of health workers in cancer (Commission of the European Communities 1986). In response to this proposal, the EU's Advisory Committee on Training in Nursing recommended that 'common training courses' in cancer nursing be developed and distributed in the different Member States (Commission of the European Communities 1988). The recommendation also proposed developments concerning education for advanced cancer nursing. In 1998, the EAC programme of the EC agreed to fund a project under the auspices of EONS to consider advanced cancer nursing practice. The project aimed to develop a framework for advanced cancer nursing practice in Europe and involved representatives from Belgium, Denmark, England, Greece, Ireland, Italy, Portugal, Scotland, Sweden and The Netherlands. As a result of individual projects undertaken in each of these countries, common themes were identified that reflect the skills, processes and anticipated outcomes of cancer nursing practice; these are presented in Box 9.4.

Identification of these themes allowed the development of a conceptual framework to support the advancement of cancer nursing practice. The framework is presented in Fig 9.1. This framework makes explicit and expands upon the necessary roles skills and processes that are required in order to advance cancer nursing practice. Fundamental to the framework is a supportive environment, which was one of the most significant factors for all the nurses wishing to advance cancer nursing practice.

■ BOX 9.4   Common themes to advance cancer nursing

Skills	Expertise, advanced knowledge, leadership, critical reflection, commitment to advancing cancer nursing practice
Processes	Networking, collaboration, facilitates change through reflection, discussion, utilization of research findings and conducting research, sets agenda for change, fosters multiprofessional working
Outcomes	Opportunities to advance cancer nursing practice, staff development and empowerment, evidence of therapeutic nursing, improved patient outcomes

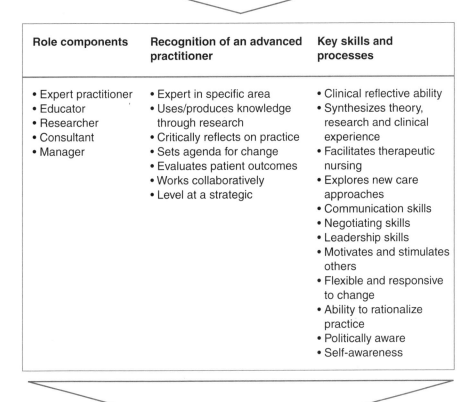

Environment to operate at an advanced level

Organizations that:
- Enable professional development
- Respect the contribution of advanced practice
- Are proactive to change
- Facilitate multiprofessional working and communication
- Are politically aware
- Are open to practitioner contribution to strategic planning

Role components	Recognition of an advanced practitioner	Key skills and processes
• Expert practitioner • Educator • Researcher • Consultant • Manager	• Expert in specific area • Uses/produces knowledge through research • Critically reflects on practice • Sets agenda for change • Evaluates patient outcomes • Works collaboratively • Level at a strategic	• Clinical reflective ability • Synthesizes theory, research and clinical experience • Facilitates therapeutic nursing • Explores new care approaches • Communication skills • Negotiating skills • Leadership skills • Motivates and stimulates others • Flexible and responsive to change • Ability to rationalize practice • Politically aware • Self-awareness

Outcomes

- Development of cancer nursing practice
- Quality patient services
- Improved patient outcomes

Figure 9.1 Conceptual framework for advanced cancer nursing practice.

Within the UK the concept of advanced nursing practice remains a much debated issue. However, there is general acceptance of the UK Central Council for Nursing and Midwifery (UKCC) statement that: 'Advanced nursing practice is concerned with adjusting the boundaries for the development of future practice, pioneering and developing new roles responsive to changing needs, and with advancing clinical practice, research and education to enrich professional practice as a whole' (UKCC 1994, p. 8). Within Europe, though, the concept of advanced nursing practice is far from clear given the diversity of professional status that is currently apparent throughout the continent. Within the context of the above project, nurse leaders from the ten European countries developed a working definition to support the need for advancing cancer nursing practice at a European level. This states: 'Advancing cancer nursing practice aims to adjust the boundaries of health care to impact patient/client outcomes. This is a dynamic innovative process demonstrated in practice and informed by education, scientific research and clinical expertise' (EONS 1999).

ADVANCING CANCER NURSING PRACTICE

In moving cancer nursing forward at a European level, the variation in culture and professional status has to be acknowledged. Therefore, any framework adopted has to be flexible enough to meet such diverse needs whilst maintaining the capacity to move the discipline forward. Developments in the next millennium in healthcare and cancer care, in particular, will challenge professionals to equate high-tech innovative treatments and care with health education and promotion and effective models for involving and supporting patients and carers in their care. In addition, nurses seek professional and academic advancement so that they may be accepted as equal members of the healthcare team. Given the developments in the profession as a whole, as outlined throughout this text, there is a changing situation and environment of care that nurses will require to work within and help to shape. Any successful framework must value and accommodate the diversity of Europe as much as its commonalities. A recent policy initiative to improve and regulate standards of care, cancer care professionals and patient outcomes in the UK may provide an effective template which may be adapted to frame the future processes of cancer care across Europe (Royal College of Nursing 1996a,b).

GOVERNMENT POLICY DIRECTIVES IN THE UK

Within the UK the Calman–Hine report (Calman & Hine 1995) described unacceptable inequalities across regional and district boundaries and sought to develop systems and processes that would minimize these inequalities and promote higher standards of cancer treatment and care. It has highlighted the importance of ensuring that the environment and culture of care are conducive to valuing staff development to enhance patient outcomes. Key recommendations from this report are outlined in Box 9.5.

There are inherent problems in the joint drive for complete equality and high expectations of high quality and service. Just as has been found in the UK, cancer care in Europe is not evenly distributed and the infrastructure available from which to provide services is very unequal, hence the tension between national or international guidelines and regional and local provision. Nevertheless, there are common issues and concerns as discussed previously which suggest that developing a lucid framework for comparison and development is appropriate and timely. Furthermore, the UK programme of standard setting and subsequent assessment has raised many issues about the role nurses can play in the

---

■ **BOX 9.5   Key recommendations from Calman & Hine (1995)**

- A new structure based on a network of expertise from primary care through cancer units to cancer centres
- Delivery of a uniform high standard of service close to people's own homes
- Cancer registries to play an important role in continuing to compile a comprehensive data set on all patients with cancer
- Adequate staff numbers to receive appropriate training and to follow identified protocols
- Services across the country to be integrated with non-cancer care and closely monitored

---

continuous monitoring of the processes and outcomes of care (Closs et al 1997, Ferguson 1997, Ferguson et al 1998).

Thus, while the context of viewing Europe and cancer nursing as one aspect of the future has changed from the early 1990s, the common themes and challenges that cancer nurses will face are more obvious. A flexible creative approach is therefore required to provide a supportive environment and to encourage nurses across country boundaries to compare and contrast the structures, cultures and outcomes of their care. The creation of practice development units may offer a suitably flexible context for peer review and development across a large number of diverse countries. This approach draws heavily on the nursing and practice development unit approach developed in the 1980s and 1990s within the UK.

THE PRACTICE DEVELOPMENT MOVEMENT IN THE UK

In the late 1980s Nursing Development Units were set up by nurses in England who sought to demonstrate the unique and holistic contribution of nurses in patient care (Malby 1996, Pearson 1983). Thereafter the Department of Health for England and Wales provided monies to support the development of 30 units within the National Health Service over 3 years, managed by the King's Fund Centre. Each unit received £30 000 per annum for development work (Redfern et al 1997).

Further evolution of this concept throughout the 1990s by the University of Leeds has resulted in the establishment of more than 60 Practice Development Units (PDUs) across England and Ireland. PDUs seek to support the development and improvement of care from a patient perspective through the creative, accountable and empowered practices of staff. These units differ from the original units in that they demonstrate the ability to develop their services and themselves within existing budgets, foster a multidisciplinary focus and include the private sector and almost every specialty of healthcare (Page et al 1998). Criteria for establishing a PDU are detailed in Box 9.6.

It became apparent in the UK implementation of its national cancer policy that, among healthcare professionals, one of nurses' greatest assets is their perceptive assessment of what will work for the patient. They come from the real world of trial and error. Often in today's drive for evidence and statistical proof, these down-to-earth skills are not valued and nurtured in the way they deserve. This is how the Leeds programme has been developed. A recent evaluation of the programme demonstrated that, where an environment is conducive to taking risk and working in creative and challenging ways, both patients and health professionals benefit (Gerrish 1999).

■ **BOX 9.6 Practice Development Unit criteria (adapted from University of Leeds 1999)**

1. A steering group that includes senior personnel representing partnerships between service and education.

2. The unit is identified as a defined area or team such as a ward, clinic, community team or primary care group.

3. The team claims ownership and accountability for the accreditation approach.

4. A PDU leader is identified who will lead the team members in the development, evaluation and dissemination of their work and will have authority for practice within the unit.

5. The team views this process of change as a positive experience.

6. The unit embraces a culture of decentralized decision-making and staff and patient empowerment.

7. Each member of the team is actively involved in personal and professional development linked to the unit's priorities.

8. The business plan includes the resources for disseminating evaluated practices both within the host organization and externally.

9. The unit operates within baseline resources comparable to other clinical care settings to enable transferability of developments.

10. Developments within the unit are evaluated in terms of their impact upon the patient, organization and staff.

11. A research-based approach to practice is developed.

12. Close collaboration with higher education enables practice to be formulated into theory.

13. The multidisciplinary team is fully involved in all developments.

14. The unit acts as a change agent within the organization, nationally and internationally publicizing its practice to promote the value of best practice.

The framework for cancer nursing services proposed here provides a structure and culture where the drive for evidence-based care prominent in Western states can be counterbalanced with the whole systems approach more common in less developed healthcare systems. These units will not only develop nursing and nurses alongside their healthcare colleagues from a practice and organizational focus, they will also encourage and support them in developing skills to lead and influence health policy (Gerrish 1999).

As stated above, nurses are often influential in their own organization but this influence does not always transcend boundaries and make an impact on the wider health agenda. PDUs can be used as training grounds for the development of both clinical and professional leadership skills (Antrobus & Kitson 1999, Christian & Norman 1998).

Clinical and professional leadership are not mutually exclusive. They have distinct characteristics. Clinical leadership is demonstrated when someone has specific clinical expertise as a core skill and works across discipline and professional boundaries in coordinating and leading expert clinical services. Professional leadership requires skills in communication, negotiation, the skilled use of power, and an element of risk-taking. Professional leaders may establish expert networks in order to inform decision-making. These principles of leadership apply to all areas of nursing. Just as cancer nurses have often led the way in new ways of thinking and working, here too they have opportunities to create new ways of working and collaborating that may inform other areas of care. The framework proposed will help nurses to become proficient in both areas of leadership.

It is important when considering the PDU structure as a basis for the framework to remember that it provides both a structure, culture and process of working that supports open ways of working and sharing. It nurtures the development of creative patient-centred practice that is evaluated and shared between and across organizational and country boundaries. In setting up a European framework for cancer nursing services, an evaluation process, built in to the planning, will map the impact of the proposed cancer care PDUs.

CONCEPTUAL FRAMEWORK FOR ADVANCING CANCER NURSING PRACTICE

The framework proposed builds on the experience and lessons learned from the nursing developments outlined above. In addition, the authors have drawn on their personal experience in developing cancer nursing both nationally and at a European level in relation to strategic development and collaborative research.

Clearly, the situation described above, in relation to developments in the UK, offers an example of a potential structure which could be adopted to develop cancer nursing at a European level. Reconstructing the environment of care within which nursing is practised is therefore fundamental to constructing a framework to advance practice. Combining the conceptual framework presented in Fig 9.1 with the concept of practice development allows the production of a framework to advance cancer nursing which could be adopted at a European level. This is presented in Fig 9.2.

The proposed framework will consist of a network of PDUs across Europe. PDUs could be supported through a range of mechanisms including leadership

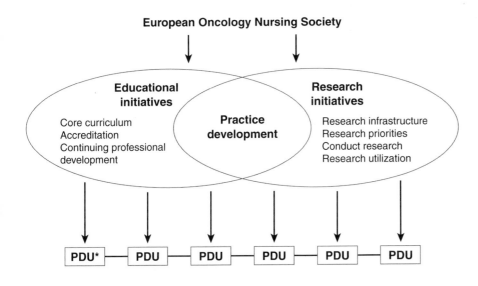

*PDU: Practice development unit

Figure 9.2 Proposed framework for European development. PDU, Practice Development Unit.

development workshops, practice monitoring, data collection, creative think-ing and working, networking and sharing, including the use of online discussion lists.

More importantly, nurse leaders involved with the PDUs would develop the skills to support the establishment and development of further units within their countries so that, through a 'train-the-trainer' process, many sites could be created within 5 years. Such a networking process enables all countries to build on their best practices and to learn from others outside their immediate sphere of experi-ence in a way that is directly related to their development of patient care and health policy rather than individual interests. The most technologically proficient countries would be no more advantaged than the rest.

With appropriate structures and cultures in place, these sites would lend them-selves easily to the further expansion of projects already developed for the collec-tion of cancer care data. They would not only provide strong clinical leadership for the sharing and development of cancer care but would enable this experience to have a wider influence on healthcare policy.

The framework would capitalize on the experience of EONS and previous work that has been undertaken in establishing PDUs, such as that described above. Clearly the project WISECARE (Kearney et al 1998) offers a template for such an ambitious project at a European level.

WISECARE stands for Workflow Information Systems for European Nursing Care and is a European Community-funded project which aims to identify the unique contribution of cancer nursing across Europe through the use of the latest information technology. To achieve this ambitious goal, WISECARE uses clinical problems to make visible the impact of cancer nursing on patient outcomes and provides a supportive network to facilitate communication and knowledge shar-ing between cancer nurses in a variety of clinical sites across Europe. WISECARE has ensured its clinical focus throughout the duration of the project by involving clinically based nurses from Scotland, Belgium, the Netherlands, Sweden and Finland.

The project has resulted in the generation of a number of products. The WISETool is a mini-electronic patient record that has been designed specifically for use within the project. It provides an integrated input–patient feedback interface for nurses and includes an instant feedback tool regarding patient outcomes for each clinical indicator. In addition, the WISECompass has been developed to mea-sure the effect of implementing the WISECARE technology on the nurses involved. The WISENet and WISEWeb are essential communication tools within the project. Other products such as the WISECARE Simulation Game, a demonstration pack-age useful for nursing education to illustrate the benefits of WISECARE technol-ogy in enhancing nursing practice, are currently under development.

In the final phase of the WISECARE project (September to December 1999), the five established clinical sites were joined by nurses in Greece, Belgium, England, Denmark, France and Slovenia. Their involvement enhanced the existing commu-nication network across Europe and their contribution facilitated the evaluation of the WISECARE project in relation to its meaningfulness in clinical practice and future use for the benefit of patients with cancer.

There can be no doubt that, in the future, healthcare will be dominated by infor-mation technology; nurses need to recognize the potential inherent within this communication medium. Any programme of development should build on exist-ing contacts and educational programmes, and utilizing the expertise developed as a result of the WISECARE programme offers cancer nurses an ideal opportunity to lead the way in advancing practice. The framework presented above offers an opportunity to realize the potential of nursing and will facilitate the accumulation of evidence as to the impact of cancer nursing on patient outcomes.

SUMMARY

This chapter has traced the development of nursing and the growing impact of cancer nursing in Europe. It has sought to outline the broad political, economic and social context in which a future strategy to develop cancer nursing must position itself. Successful European precedents for collaboration and joint education and advancement have been highlighted. It is hoped that the ideas presented here will serve as the basis for the growth of an incremental strategy for cancer nursing across Europe that is created and moulded by the readers of this book and their colleagues in cancer care.

REFERENCES

Antrobus S, Kitson A 1999 Nursing leadership: influencing and shaping health policy and nursing practice. Journal of Advanced Nursing 29(3):746–753

Asvall J 1997 Foreword. In: Salvage J & Heijen S (eds) Nursing in Europe: a resource for better health. WHO Regional Publications, European Series No 74, Geneva, p xiii

Bond P, Jodrell N 1997 Cancer nursing in Europe: an account based on interviews with students, nurses and doctors. Journal of Cancer Nursing 1(2):81–85

Calman K, Hine D 1995 A commissioning framework for cancer services. NHS Executive, London

Carroll S, 1998 Role of the breast care clinical nurse specialist in facilitating decision-making for treatment choice: a practice profile. European Journal of Oncology Nursing 2(1):34–42

Christian S, Norman I 1998 Clinical leadership in nursing development units. Journal of Advanced Nursing 27:108–116

Closs S J, Ferguson A, Rae M J 1997 Developing local cancer nursing services in the wake of a national policy. Journal of Cancer Nursing 1(1):16–24

Commission of the European Communities 1986 'Europe Against Cancer' programme: proposal for a plan of action 1987–1989. Commission of the European Communities (COM 86/717 final), Luxembourg

Commission of the European Communities 1988 Advisory Committee on Training in Nursing: report and recommendations on training in cancer. Commission of the European Communities III/D/248/3/88-EN, Brussels

Corner J 1991 Cancer nursing in Europe: beyond 2000. European Journal of Cancer Care 1(1):11–14

Corner J 1995 Innovative approaches in symptom management. European Journal of Cancer Care 4(4):145–146

European Oncology Nursing Society 1990 A core curriculum for a postbasic course in cancer nursing. Cancer Nursing 13(2):123–128

European Oncology Nursing Society 1999 Advanced cancer nursing practice/standards project final report. Project number 96/CAN/35236. Europe Against Cancer Programme, European Commission, Luxembourg

European Union Publication (1997a) Annual report on equal opportunities between men and women. Social Europe Series. EU, Brussels

European Union Publication 1997b Work and childcare – a guide to good practice. Social Europe Series. EU, Brussels

Ferguson A 1997 Cancer services: investing for the future. Department of Health and Social Services, Belfort, Northern Ireland

Ferguson A, Makin W, Walker B, Dublon G 1998 Regional implementation of a national cancer policy: taking forward multiprofessional collaborative cancer care. European Journal of Cancer Care 7(3):162–167

Gerrish K 1999 An evaluation of the practice development programme at the Centre for the Development of Nursing Policy and Practice at the University of Leeds. CDNPP, University of Leeds, Leeds

Jodrell N 1997 An assessment of the activities in the area of training in oncology for nurses, Europe Against Cancer programme project no. 96/CAN/47281. European Commission, Luxembourg

Kearney N, Campbell S, Sermeus W 1998 Practising for the future: utilising information technology in cancer nursing practice. European Journal of Oncology Nursing 2(3):169–175

Knowles G, Kearney N 1998 Advancing cancer nursing practice in Europe: an overview. European Journal of Oncology Nursing 2(3):156–161

Ludvigsen C, Roberts K 1996 Health care policies and Europe – the implications for practice. Butterworth-Heinemann, Oxford

Malby R 1996 Nursing Development Units in the United Kingdom. Advanced Practice Nursing Quarterly 1(4):20–27

Page S, Allsop D & Casley S (eds) 1998 The Practice Development Unit – an experiment in multidisciplinary innovation. Whurr, London

Patiraki-Kourbani E, Lanara V, Monos D, Ifantopoulos J, Mantas J, Plati C 1998 Nursing assessment of pain in cancer patients: the Greek picture. European Journal of Oncology Nursing 2(2):133–135

Pearson A 1983 The clinical nursing unit. Heinemann, London

Redfern S, Normand C, Christian S, Gilmore A, Murrels T, Norman I, Stevens W 1997 An evaluation of nursing development units. NT Research 2(4):292–303

Royal College of Nursing 1996a A structure for cancer nursing. Cancer Nursing Society, London

Royal College of Nursing 1996b Guidelines for good practice in cancer nursing education. Cancer Nursing Society, London

Salvage J 1993 Raising the nursing profile: the case of the invisible nurse. World Health Statistics Quarterly 46(3):170–176

Salvage J 1998 Nursing on the European map. Nursing Times 94(6):55–58

Salvage J, Heijnen S 1997 Nursing in Europe: a resource for better health. World Health Organization European Series No. 74, WHO, Copenhagen

United Kingdom Central Council for Nursing and Midwifery 1994 The future of professional practice – the Council's standards for education and practice following registration. Position Statement on Policy Implementation. UKCC, London

University of Leeds 1999 Practice development criteria. Centre for the Development of Nursing Policy and Practice, University of Leeds, Leeds

World Bank 1993 Investing in health; the World Bank development report. World Bank, New York

Index